Florian Steger

Asclepius
Medicine and Cult

Translated from the German by Margot M. Saar

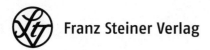 Franz Steiner Verlag

Bibliographic information published by the German National Library:
The German National Library lists this publication in the Deutsche Nationalbiblio-
grafie; detailed bibliographic information is available at <http://dnb.d-nb.de>.

© Franz Steiner Verlag, Stuttgart 2018
Druck: Hubert & Co., Göttingen
Gedruckt auf säurefreiem, alterungsbeständigem Papier.
Printed in Germany.
ISBN 978-3-515-12197-2 (Print)
ISBN 978-3-515-12201-6 (E-Book)

Contents

Preface

This book is a translated and revised version of my former "Asklepios: Medizin und Kult" (STEGER 2016a) and is published in answer to many and frequent requests from various sides. Any literature published since 2016 has been added throughout the text. A section on the *Iamatica* of Poseidippus has been added to chapter III.3. Three figures have been added, one has been exchanged. Critical comments in reviews published so far on STEGER (2016a) have been considered. Again, I have to thank Dr. Frank Ursin, who is a faithful and wise companion of my research in medical history, especially in the field of ancient medicine. Furthermore I thank Margot M. Saar for her translation of the manuscript. Last but not least I thank Dr. Thomas Schaber for his support of my research into Asclepius.

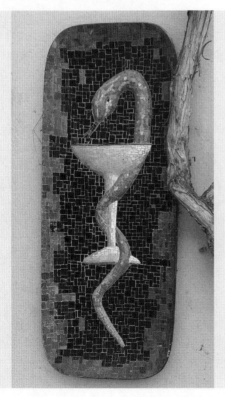

Fig. 1 – Serpent of Asclepius, mosaic, Lindau (Germany)

I

Introduction

Everyday life is determined by biological phenomena such as birth, life and death, and, as biological processes, health and illness impact importantly on the way people live. With a few exceptions, most people do what they can to preserve their health and combat illness. A look at the history of cultures reveals a wide variety of health-related problems and conditions, approaches and applications (PORTER 2000 and GRMEK 1989).

It was in the course of the Roman imperial period that a consciousness of health- and illness-related problems gradually emerged, and with it a colorful array of healthcare providers: sorcerers and miracle workers representing a magic-demonic approach, healing cults offering theurgic rituals and healing concepts, midwives and drug-dealers, each of them constituting a non-medical group that operated, however, in close proximity to the scientific medical practitioners. And each of them was in itself highly heterogeneous: the physicians, for instance, can be divided into private, public and military practitioners. For any groups that did not produce written records of their experiences, other sources need to be consulted. GUMMERUS (1932) and OEHLER (1909) have collected epigraphic testimonies to public and private physicians as representatives of scientific medicine, HILLERT (1990) and JACKSON (1988: 56–85) have assembled archaeological evidence. While there are publications on the military physicians (e. g. SAMAMA 2017), research on private and public physicians are surprisingly few and far between, a fact that is partly due to the sources being widely dispersed. In contrast to the knowledge we have of physicians who were also writers (such as Celsus or Galen), information on individual – male or female – medical practitioners is fairly sparse.

As a whole, these groups provided a multifaceted market of healthcare and healing approaches that contributed significantly to the cultural life in general. Efforts were made, moreover, to place medicine on solid theoretical foundations, an endeavor that was, as the contemporary specialist literature reveals, surrounded by some controversy.

Research into ancient medicine, which is mostly conducted by classical philologists, tends to concentrate on this specialist literature, of which the Hippocratic Corpus and the works of Galen of Pergamum and Aulus Cornelius Celsus constitute the keystones. And yet, it must be borne in mind that any conclusions regarding the actual practice of medicine that can be derived from these sources are of limited validity. The same is true for the medical knowledge of the Islamic Golden Age, which has always been based on Avicenna's *Canon Medicinae*. This *princeps medicorum* has been assigned a central place in medieval medicine but little consideration has been given to the fact that he represented only one of many approaches to medicine in the caliphate (STROHMAIER 1999 and WEISSER 1983).

The affiliation of religion and medicine, which is manifest in the healing cults above all, presents as a separate field of research. Among the most important of these ritual, cultic forms of healing was the cult surrounding the hero and later god of healing, Asclepius, who was called Aesculapius by the Romans. From the fourth century BCE, magnificent temples (*Asclepieia*) were dedicated to Asclepius all across the Mediterranean world and further afield, in Gallia and Germania. In these temples Asclepius was worshipped and there, those seeking healing for their ailments would find help. This book will demonstrate how the healing cult of Asclepius, the god of healing, provided a particular form of medicine that encompassed more than its defining, and important, religious elements. The medicine of Asclepius was practiced in his temples and, with its interweaving of cult and medicine that will need to be examined in more depth, it was an important element of the healthcare on offer in the Roman Empire. KRUG (1993: 141) points out correctly that the research literature does, for the most part, not assign particular importance to this form of treatment. And yet, such lack of recognition seems unwarranted, historically as well as medically – as will be illustrated in chapter III.5, which examines some inscriptions from this cult, giving particular emphasis to medical-historical analysis.

—

Research has focused primarily on the religious and mythical aspects of the Asclepian healing cult, but its medical elements, and consequently its position within the history of medicine, have been of equal interest. Scientists have tried above all to ascertain where between the religious-magic and the scientific-rational approaches to healing the medicine of Asclepius is to be located. The thesis of a separate Asclepian medicine that had fused with the healing cult whilst continuing to be informed by a scientific-rational approach and relying on observation and an understanding of nature has so far been largely discounted. If at all, such developments have been assigned to the Roman imperial period, but no arguments have as yet been brought forward that could give weight to this view.

An older publication by EDELSTEIN/EDELSTEIN, consisting of two comprehensive volumes, contains almost all the written sources on Asclepius available up to 1945. Volume I presents these sources in their original language and in English translation, with annotations, while Volume II offers an overall evaluation (both parts were newly published in one volume in 1998). Interpretation based on this material alone is, on the whole, restricted to the mythological aspects and the cult's religious-historical significance, an approach that was pursued before by OHLEMUTZ (1940) and WEINREICH (1909). This interpretation, which focuses on the fifth and fourth centuries BCE, is no longer in keeping with modern-day methods of epigraphic evaluation. The stone inscriptions that have been preserved only reflect some of the materials commonly used for epigraphy – others were wood, fabric, and leather – and are therefore not fully representative (ECK 1997: 95–98).

In most cases only the sources themselves are interpreted but they are neither contextualized during analysis nor interrogated as to their representative strength. Another aspect that remains unconsidered is that the epigrams themselves only record what was intended to be preserved for posterity. EDELSTEIN/EDELSTEIN failed to recognize the division that comes to light when one reads through their collection of testimonies, and that calls attention to a new development in the medicine and cult of Asclepius, starting with the first century BCE. The sources collated by EDELSTEIN/EDELSTEIN therefore need to be critically re-evaluated with the inclusion of any findings from after 1945.

LIDONNICI (1995) – and PEEK before her, in 1993 – presented a new and annotated text edition on the Epidaurian stele inscriptions (IG IV² 1.121–124). She examined three Epidaurian epigraphs, plus fragments of a fourth, which are known from PAUSANIAS (2.27.3) and go back to the (late) second half of the fourth century BCE, and published them with individual annotations in the original as well as in English translation. The new collection of sources by GIRONE (1998) is worth mentioning, too, because it includes further imperial epigraphs. In a selection of examples, which seems somewhat arbitrary, GIRONE brings together 32 individually annotated epigraphs from Athens, Epidaurus, Lebena, Pergamum and Rome, all originating in the period between the fourth century BCE and the fourth century CE. Missing from this publication are an overall assessment in addition to the individual comments and (as was the case with EDELSTEIN/EDELSTEIN also) the inclusion of sources other than inscriptions.

Unlike EDELSTEIN/EDELSTEIN, LIDONNICI, and GIRONE, KRUG (1993:120–187) not only includes the written sources, but gives equal consideration to the numismatic and archaeological testimonies, making her comprehensive chapter on Asclepius therefore a, so far, unique evaluation of the Asclepius material. After introducing the Asclepian myth and its representations, KRUG describes the healing cult and the individual locations where it flourished, including those in Britannia and Hispania, and concludes that Asclepius was entrusted with the healthcare and welfare of all sick people. She contends that this makes Asclepius the refuge of the unhealed who had been turned away elsewhere because, in accordance with Hippocratic tradition (De Arte 3 (6.4.16–6.6.1 L.)), physicians refused to treat patients who were considered incurable (VON STADEN 1990 and WITTERN 1979).

Asclepius was also able to cure aspects of afflictions that were not accessible to rational explanation. In contrast to EDELSTEIN/EDELSTEIN, KRUG (1993: 121) sees Asclepius' medical interventions as complementary since the periods when Asclepius flourished were contemporaneous with the highpoints of medicine. NUTTON (2004: 114) contended therefore that Hippocratic medicine and the cult of Asclepius together formed an alternative to magic medicine on the ancient health market. A closer investigation into practicing physicians is missing, however, and so the question as to the relationship they had with the Asclepieia remains open. KRUG relies instead on the writings of the Hippocratic tradition, although COHN-HAFT (1956: 29–31) and JACKSON (1988: 140) had already concluded that relationships between practicing physicians and the Asclepian healing sites had existed since the fourth century BCE. WICKKISER (2008) even asserted such a relationship for the fifth century BCE, but is unable to present convincing evidence to corroborate this theory.

SCHNALKE/WITTERN (1993) and SCHNALKE (1990: 1–35) largely agree with KRUG's view and consequently refrain from differentiating between an Asclepian cult and Asclepian medicine. They hold instead that the rise of Asclepius occurred to compensate for the gradual repression of magic-mystical approaches (SCHNALKE/WITTERN 1993: 89). This view is opposed to that of the Hippocrates expert JOUANNA (1996: 48 f.) who saw the religious healing practiced in the Asclepian temples as distinct from medicine. SCHNALKE/WITTERN (1993: 100), on the other hand – in opposition to EDELSTEIN/EDELSTEIN and KRUG – detect a clear division between the Asclepian treatments used in classical Greece and those of the Roman imperial period. In agreement with JACKSON (1988: 138–169), and opposing the view of SCARBOROUGH (1696: 24 f.), they claim that the medical treatments provided in the imperial *Asclepieia* were rational and scientific. Earlier investigations into the medicine on offer in the Asclepieia during the imperial period were carried out by HAHN (1976) and MÜLLER (1987).

HAEHLING VON LANZENAUER (1996) focused less on the medicine in her dissertation and more on the cult of Asclepius, as RÜTTIMANN had done earlier (1986) in a religious-historical investigation based on a similar research question. It is the central role they both assign to the aspect of healing (Asclepius Soter – Imperator soter – Christus Soter) that makes their work interesting for our investigation. They consider the alliance between imperial cult and Asclepian piety to have been a genuine threat to Christianity. As healers, both the Princeps and Asclepius were confronting Christ the healer. The imperial cult tried to exploit the pious dedication to Asclepius and it is therefore conceivable that, after Constantine, the cult of Asclepius was deliberately expanded and instrumentalized, even though the Christian faith was prevailing over the pagan cults at that time. Focusing on the cult of Asclepius in the second century CE, RÜTTIMANN (1986) makes an even more compelling case for the view that the worshippers of Asclepius – just like the Christians, and guided by similar theological considerations – saw miraculous cures as a proof of divinity. The cult of Asclepius therefore retained its importance while other pagan cults began to fade away. It can therefore be concluded that Asclepius did not make way for his Christian rival until the end of the ancient period, and not without having left his imprint on its approach to healing.

HART (2000) has knowledgeably compiled the wide array of sources available in relation to Asclepius, the god of medicine. His volume is richly adorned with images that often succeed in creating a link to the present but also lend the work an air of popular science. HART, moreover, restricts himself to the older work by EDELSTEIN/EDELSTEIN (1945) as the inspiration for his monograph. Any research conducted after 1945 is only included marginally and selectively, and once again, the old thesis is aired that the only patients to turn to Asclepius were those whom the physicians were unable to cure; that their afflictions were mostly psychosomatic and that Asclepius was able to offer them a therapy with placebo effect (HART 2000: 89) – a thesis that is not convincing in the historically undifferentiated form in which it is presented.

This outline of the overall research situation reveals an obvious gap: Asclepius research so far has focused on aspects of religious history but has not taken into account the medical dimension. The development of Asclepian medicine from its beginnings in the fifth century BCE up until the Roman imperial period has not been documented convincingly and it therefore remains uncertain how medicine was integrated into the cultic rituals. Researchers rarely differentiate between the cult of Asclepius and the medicine of Asclepius, and no one has as yet thought of considering the medicine of Asclepius as an integral part of the Roman Empire's medical culture. The epigraphic, numismatic, and archaeological sources providing evidence of this culture have been evaluated by RIETHMÜLLER (2005), but his extensive research material is difficult to use because of the way it is structured. An exemplary contribution has been made by the Italian MELFI (2007), who carried out in-depth research into the major and minor *Asclepieia* on the Peloponnese, the Cyclades, and in Central Greece. And yet, neither of these works manages to convey a clear picture of Asclepian medicine.

Systematic assessments of the epigraphic material have so far been attempted by BENEDUM (1977), PFOHL (1977), ROWLAND (1977), NUTTON (1977/1972/1970/1969), COHN-HAFT (1956), GUMMERUS (1932), HABERLING (1910), OEHLER (1909) and POHL (1905). The numismatic testimonies have mostly been investigated in scattered specialist researches undertaken by AGELIDIS (1911), SZAIVERT (2008), and KRANZ (2004), to name but a few, on Pergamum, and by HAYMANN (2010) on Aegeae. KAMPMANN (1993) studied the imperial coins in relation to Asclepius, and PENN (1994) examined Greek and Roman coins and their references to medicine in general.

This monograph aims to delineate the medicine of Asclepius in as much detail as possible based on the scattered sources available on imperial medicine. Historically, it focuses on the Roman imperial period (27 BCE to 284 CE). Earlier or later sources will also be taken into account as long as they facilitate a better understanding of the subject under consideration. Presenting the rituals performed in the *Asclepieia* as an integral part of the eclectic healing market of that cultural period will add another dimension to the research into the cult of Asclepius, which has so far been restricted to aspects of religious history; it will, moreover, illustrate how important a role the medicine of Asclepius played within that context. As a first step it will be necessary to provide a portrait of everyday life during the period in question, in which the cult and medicine of Asclepius can be embedded. Using primarily inscriptions for this investigation seems appropriate seeing that the first and second centuries CE have been designated the "era of epigraphic culture" (ECK 1997: 99). Dedicatory inscriptions prove most useful in this undertaking because they express the gratitude visitors felt toward Asclepius, reflect the piety and trust of the worshippers, and, in some cases, contain descriptions of the healing process itself. Also included will be funerary inscriptions for physicians, which may provide insights into the medical profession and activities, as well as honorific inscriptions to physicians, which often reflect the benefactor's own love for self-presentation. 525 inscriptions of Greek physicians have been gathered by SAMAMA (2003). In all this it needs to be borne in mind that – however valuable the epigraphic testimonies are – they only record what was intended for commemoration. Their representative value therefore is to be critically scrutinized and it is clear that this investigation cannot rely on inscriptions alone; but neither must the epigraphic material be discounted altogether, as it was by EDELSTEIN/EDELSTEIN (1945). The route that recommends itself is to use the inscriptions and complement them with evaluations of the relevant literature, the numismatic and archaeological sources, and the papyri.

The author proposes that during the Roman imperial period the medicine of Asclepius contributed significantly to the healthcare market by offering a complex web of therapies. The medicine practiced in the Asclepian sanctuaries consisted in a combination of cultic healing rituals and medical therapies. The productive interweaving of cult and medicine that characterizes it gives it its undoubted place as part of the healthcare market in the Roman Empire.

This book will first introduce the wide range of imperial healthcare available (II), and then use this as a foundation for arguing in favor of an independent Asclepian medicine. The eclectic nature of the healthcare on offer during the imperial period (II.1) derives from a cultural and historical development that can be traced back to the ancient orient and from there to Greece. These cultural origins are mentioned if they can support the main thesis (II.2). A review of the cultural history reveals that the practice of medicine has always gone hand in hand with the endeavor to underpin this practice with solid theoretical foundations. An introduction to the medical theory (II.3) that arose from, and at the same time influenced, the medical practice is therefore essential for an understanding of everyday healthcare and medicine. It is important to note that independent traditions with large numbers of followers need to be distinguished from individuals who, in some cases, also kept written records (II.4). The varied groups providing practical everyday healthcare (II.5) included physicians, midwives and drug-dealers (who were not considered medical practitioners), and representatives of magic and religious cults. All together these groups offered a wide array of health services that is enriched by the inclusion of Asclepian medicine (III). Asclepius, the hero and later god of healing, was very popular and highly revered and his healing cult is no less important than those of Heracles or Serapis (III.1). Between the fourth century BCE and the sixth century CE the Asclepian healing cult became so prominent and influential that it grew far beyond the Mediterranean world. Thanks to the devotion of his worshippers, Asclepius, the pagan god of healing, was able to hold his own for a long time alongside the Christian god.

Cultic rituals were performed in special sanctuaries dedicated to Asclepius. Those afflicted with illness also came to these sacred places, where they prayed to Asclepius for healing. These sites of Asclepian practice (III.2) can be further investigated as to their social function and particularly also their location and layout. Another interesting question is how the devotees spent their time in these sanctuaries: where they stayed, where they had contact with Asclepius, where the therapy took place, and what kind of measures or facilities enhanced their experience inside the sanctuary. On examination of individual cases it can be demonstrated to what extent healing was experienced solely as a result of Asclepius appearing to patients in their dreams, in a fashion similar to that of reported miracles in the Christian tradition (III.3), or whether rational instructions were also conveyed to these patients. The author will attempt to look at the healing processes experienced in the Asclepian temples "bottom up", that is from the patient's perspective. Aelius Aristides, who is renowned for his literary work, left such introspective reports which grant deeper insights into the medical provision at Pergamum (III.5.1). In addition there are inscriptions that also describe healing processes. Two patients, one who attended the sanctuary in Epidaurus (III.5.2) and another who went to the temple at Pergamum (III.5.3), use such inscriptions to relate their experiences of Asclepian medicine. In conjunction with the topographical accounts of the Asclepian temples these reports convey a good picture of the entire healing procedure. Against this background of the daily medical practice it is possible to gain an understanding of the myth surrounding Asclepius, of his healing cult and, above all, of his medicine during the Roman imperial period.

II

The Medicine of Asclepius in Context

II.1 – The beginnings of the Asclepian cult in Rome

As early as the Republic if not even earlier, during the Kingdom, Rome boasted a healthcare market that was sustained by a heterogeneous array of healers. The healthcare provision available extended from magical approaches to healing cults to medical activities in the narrower sense. The impulses leading to the establishment of such a unique and diverse market came with the growing urbanization and trade, both of which facilitated cultural transfer. The Etruscans, Greeks, the peoples of Southern Italy, and the Phoenicians, who brought with them the wisdom of Egypt (HELCK 1995 and BURKERT 1984), entertained a lively exchange with Rome and the growing Roman Empire.

The first contact with Greek healing occurred via the cult of Apollo when, in 433 BCE, the Romans vowed to erect a temple to this deity, hoping that he would protect them from the plague that was sweeping through the country (LIV. 4.25). Up until Augustan times, this remained the only temple in Rome that was dedicated to Apollo. But although *Apollo Medicus* (BECHER 1970: 214–216) had been acknowledged ever since Hesiod as the father of Asclepius (PAUS. 2.26.7), and although he had the power to inflict and remove illness (HOM. II. 1.42–53), this was not the beginning of the healing tradition, on the one hand because it was a very primitive cult and, on the other, because no Greek priests had accompanied it to Rome (for an opposing view cf. SCARBOROUGH 1969: 24 f.).

It was none less than Asclepius, the Greek god of healing, whose arrival in Rome in 293 BCE heralded the dawn of Rome's medical history (LIV. 1.47, AUG. civ. 3.12 and 3.17, PLIN. nat. 29.16). Ancient numismatic depictions (fig. 2) reveal that a sanctuary was consecrated to Asclepius two years later on Tiber Island, marking the beginning of a Rome's vibrant coexistence and interaction of foreign cultures in Rome.

Soon the first medical traders arrived. The first Greek physician in Rome was Archagathus who arrived in 218 BCE (PLIN. nat. 29.12). Asclepiades of Prusa ad Mare in Bithynia needs to be mentioned, too, because he reintroduced Greek medicine in Rome around 90 BCE and went down in history as the innovator of Roman Medicine (PLIN. nat. 7.123 f. and 26.12–20, and VALLANCE 1993/1990). Cato the Elder, Varro, and Pliny the Elder, who disseminated a kind of family medicine, were replaced by medical specialists, some of whom left their specialist writings to posterity in a development that rang in profound changes.

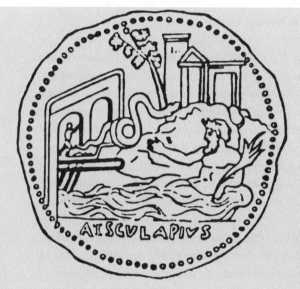

Fig. 2 – Medallion of Antoninus Pius: the serpent of Asclepius arrives on Tiber Island

While the cult of Asclepius was a Greek import for the Romans, its place of origin continues to be controversially discussed by researchers, the alternatives under consideration being Trikka in Thessaly (today's Trikala) and Epidaurus on the Peloponnese. The early Homeric references point to Epidaurus, but the explicit statements of the Augustan geographer Strabo speak for Trikka. Neither of these views has so far been corroborated by archaeological excavations (III.1).

II.2 – Relations with Ancient Babylon and Egypt

The cultural encounter between ancient Hellas and ancient Babylon in which dogs appear to be a common motif proves that the cultural roots of Asclepius reach far beyond mainland Greece (LORENZ 2004/2016 and BURKERT 1984: 75–77). PAUSANIAS (2.27.2) speaks of an image made of gold and ivory that was exhibited in the temple of Asclepius at Epidaurus. This image shows Asclepius with a dog stretched out next to him. According to AELIAN (nat. 7.13), sacred dogs once protected the Asclepieion in Athens against a thief. The sanctuary of *Apollo Maleatas* (whose heir Asclepius was) stood on Mount Kynortion, a name that also contains a reference to dogs (LORENZ 2000: 211 f.). A further canine reference appears in a votive relief that depicts the two sons of Asclepius, Podalirius and Machaon, accompanied by a dog (KERÉNYI 1956: fig. 15 and HAUSMANN 1948: fig. 10). According to the myth Asclepius was nursed by a dog after his abandonment on Mount Kynortion, where he was later found by dog handlers (APOLLOD. FGrHist 244 F 138); and dogs are mentioned again in the *lex sacra,* an inscription discovered in Piraeus, which mentions preliminary sacrificial offerings to Maleatas, Apollo, Hermes, Jason, Aceso, Panacea, and to dogs and dog handlers (IG II/III² 4962).

There clearly was an intimate connection between Asclepius and dogs, and dogs were also associated with healing in ancient Babylon (LORENZ 2000: 260–266). Three small bronze figurines, which were found in the sanctuary of Hera in Samos and which depict a praying man with a dog, refer to Gula of Isin, the Babylonian goddess of healing also known as *azugallatu,* the great healer (LORENZ 1988: 5 f. and KYRIELEIS 1979). Gula was as ambivalent a deity of healing as Apollo because she, too, could inflict and cure illness (MAUL 2001: 20 and AVALOS 1995: 99–232).

The noticeable ubiquity of images depicting Asclepius in the company of a dog may be an indication that a familiar image had been imported from ancient Babylon, with the dog symbolizing the canine sacrifices common in the cult of Gula of Isin, the great healer (*azugallatu*), who is always portrayed with dogs. There is evidence of countless dog burials in her temple which, judging by the many (mostly anatomical) votive offerings discovered there, was clearly a place of pilgrimage.

Not only Asclepius, but his mythical father, Apollo, too, is connected with the Babylonian healing cult (HOM. Hymn. 16). On the Cycladic island of Anafi, near Thiry, Apollo was venerated as Ἀσγελάτας (Asgelatas) (IG XII 3,248 f.). Phonetically, Ἀσγελάτας is identical with *azugallatu,* the epithet assigned to Gula, the Babylonian goddess of healing. In Anafi, Apollo was consequently referred to as Ἀσγελάτας and worshipped as a physician, which corresponds to one of his most important functions (ARISTOPH. Av. 584: Apollon Iatros). There is also evidence that dogs and puppies were present in the temples of Astarte and Mukol in the Cyprian city of Kition. The fact that in Idalion on Cyprus, where he bore the epithet of Amuklos, Apollo was equated with Resheph-Mukol accounts for yet another association with dogs (LORENZ

2000: 266). Apollo, his son Asclepius and the sons of Asclepius are, through their titles and the way they are portrayed, associated with Gula of Isin, the Babylonian goddess of healing, and it is therefore difficult to deny that both Asclepius and Apollo have roots that go back all the way to ancient Babylon.

As in the case of Mesopotamian medicine, Asclepius again builds the bridge between Egyptian and Hellenic healing cults. He is associated with the healing cult of Imhotep (third millennium BCE; RENBERG 2017: 456–466, ŁAJTAR 2006 *and* LORENZ 1988: 5 f.), who, as far as one can tell today, was not a physician and was not elevated to demigod status until after his death, in the Persian period (KOLTA/SCHWARZMANN-SCHAFHAUSER 2000: 72–78). He was a lector-priest to King Djoser (around 2600 BCE) as well as a renowned architect. His role as a healing hero included caring for the sick and promoting fertility. Asclepius and Imhotep share the way in which they bring healing. For both of them incubation and dream appearances, in which they imparted diagnostic and therapeutic information to the patients, were of great importance (RENBERG 2017: 115–270 and 448–483).

II.3 – Medical Traditions

The meeting of Roman and Greek cultures led to the formation of separate medical traditions, each of which had its own practicing physicians. There was, for instance, the eclectic group of *Dogmatists* whose approach was based on the old tradition of a rational medicine. They believed that illnesses had hidden as well as evident causes and that therapies often started with guesswork. The second group, the *Empiricists*, rejected the idea of covert causes because in their view one can only understand what one perceives with one's senses. For them, medicine was based on experience. The third group, the *Methodists*, was central to the imperial period. Like the *Empiricists*, they refused to acknowledge hidden causes. Influenced by the ideas of Asclepiades of Bithynia, they put forward their own medical theory, in which the triad of phenomenon, commonality, and indication played a prominent part. In addition to these three traditions, which were described by Celsus in that order, there were the *Pneumatists* who thought that the *pneuma* (literally 'breath' or 'soul'), from which the world fashioned the human body, revealed itself in the pulse. The fifth and final group, known as the *Anonymous*, subscribed to the ideas of humoral pathology, extended by a localized notion of illness.

Celsus explained in his proem to *De arte medicina* that, in Rome, three separate groups could be differentiated on the basis of their approach to medicine: Dogmatists, Empiricists, and Methodists (CELS. pr. 12). Scientists refer to these groups as medical 'schools'. In doing so they adopt the classification put forward in the medical textbooks of the Roman and Byzantine periods and promote the later canonization in the Middle Ages (BÜHLER/COHNITZ 2005). The term 'school' goes back to the concept of the medical sect (*secta*), for which there is no evidence until the third century BCE in Alexandria (VON STADEN 1989/1982). Herophilus, a physician who hailed from Bithynia (born around 330 BCE in Chalcedon, PS.-GAL. Introduct. 14.683 K.) paved the way for such a group in Alexandria by gathering a group of pupils around him. Among these pupils were Philinus of Cos, who would later lead the *Empiricists*, and Bacchius of Tanagra. This kind of group – called αἵρεσις (*hairesis*) in Greek and *secta* or *factio* in Latin, depended on a teacher who would teach his tenets to a circle of students. The students would be expected to accept these teachings and protect them against attacks from outside, by followers of other traditions for instance. While there is evidence enough to testify to the existence of such approaches, it is difficult to assess with any certainty how influential each of them was (LEITH 2016 and GOUREVITCH 1996: 114–117). Celsus mentioned the three subgroups for the first time in his proem; he does, however, not speak explicitly of 'schools' either but of '*partes*' (parties), a term that suggests something like a political group. It is difficult to identify three such groups because later tradition adopted the system suggested by Celsus. The term 'school' is consequently a didactic categorization and it is more appropriate to speak of traditions (SELINGER 1999: 34).

Celsus divided the groups according to the way they acquired their knowledge. The dogmatic tradition, which is linked to Hippocrates of Cos (LABISCH 2005a, and SCHUBERT 2005: 61–66), sees science as the study of what is observed most commonly in more or less the same way and strives to verify the findings of rationalistic medicine by means of anatomical insights. The dissecting of human corpses is essential for this approach (CELS. pr. 23 f. and SELINGER 1999: 35 f.). Two further, very prominent groups are those around Herophilus and Erasistratus. The latter descended from a family of physicians in Ioulis on the island of Ceos (SMITH 1982 and FRASER 1969). He continued the work of Herophilus and also conducted vivisections. Both are seen as the founders of Western human anatomy.

Up to that point, anatomy had been restricted to the dissection of animals for ethical and religious reasons (LORENZ 2000: 186–190, SELINGER 1990: 30, WITTERN 1999: 552, and WITTERN 1995: 21–30). Then suddenly, not only human corpses were dissected but vivisections were carried out on convicted criminals (SELINGER 1999: 37–39 and VON STADEN 1989: 138–153). This development slowed down after Erasistratus but was newly stimulated by Galen.

While there is evidence of continuing human dissections in the Byzantine east, there was no dissection of humans in the west until the late thirteenth century CE (Wittern 1999/1998a).

In his proem CELSUS presents the main characteristics of the dogmatic tradition in distinction to its rival approaches (pr. 13–26): obscure causes of an illness can be penetrated by the physician who will then try to derive an etiology from them. In addition to the hidden causes, he describes evident, sense-perceptible causes. Illness is directly preceded by cold or heat, hunger or satiety. Anatomical and physiological complications can be resolved by logical thinking. The dogmatic tradition is informed by differentiated notions regarding individual bodily structures and their interaction. Therapies are chosen by conjecture, using the hidden cause as an indicator. Dissections can supply important additional information and experience which can be meaningfully applied in therapy.

Philinus of Cos was the first to oppose these ideas. As a pupil of Herophilus he started off as a Dogmatist but later he broke with his teacher and his view of medicine. At around 250 BCE he introduced the *Empiricist* tradition in Alexandria. This tradition is seen as the oldest because according to Pliny (nat. 29.5) it was founded around 430 BCE by Acron of Acragas in Sicily (GUARDASOLE 2005 and DEICHGRÄBER 1948: fr. 5–7). Its principal underlying precept is that nothing can be understood that cannot be perceived with the senses. For the *Empiricists* medicine is therefore – as their name suggests – determined by experience. An actual medical theory that could be passed on from teacher to pupil cannot be derived from this approach. This tradition is therefore a good example of the doubtfulness of the term "school" in this context (Nutton 1997: 1016). According to the *Empiricists*, illness is indicated by symptoms that are perceptible to the senses. Because nature is comprehensible and real, the hidden causes assumed by the *Dogmatists* can have no reality. Experiments were consequently not needed to enhance understanding and vivisections or autopsies were futile. The *Empiricists* believed that the medical practice and treatment of patients offered sufficient opportunities for gaining knowledge on the provision of healthcare. Treatment was based on conclusions from analogy and similarity between cases determined the choice of therapy. For the same reason knowledge gained from books played a particular part in this approach to medicine.

Apart from the *Dogmatists* and the *Empiricists* there were the *Methodists*. In addition to Celsus' proem, we also have information from Soranus of Ephesus about this tradition of which he was a representative (LABISCH 2005b and MEISSNER 1999: 219–221). With his encyclopedic writings on practical training, Soranus established gynecology as a medical specialization with its own literature. We also learn much about the *Methodist* tradition indirectly from Caelius Aurelianus, who preserved one of Soranus' lost works in Latin translation in *Celerum sive acutarum passionum* and *Tardarum sive chronicarum passionum* (MEISSNER 1999: 309, incl. note 737).

The *Methodist* tradition is very important to the imperial period (CELS. pr. 54 with PIGEAUD 1982 and MEYER-STEINEG 1916). To some extent it built on the *Empiricist* tradition, for instance in showing the same lack of interest in hidden causes; but it also drew on the thinking of Asclepiades of Bithynia. Lastly, it had, like the dogmatic tradition, its own theoretical view and claimed that knowledge arose from, drew upon and perpetuated previously existing insights. The *Methodists* actively transformed knowledge, imbuing it with their own cultural views. The Methodist tradition was no established science but rather a body of knowledge that constantly needed to be adjusted and was therefore always in flux. Its representatives were not looking for hidden causes nor were they pure *Empiricists*. It must be assumed that the *Methodists* were critical of the *Dogmatists* because of their practice of vivisection. The triad of phenomenon, commonality, and indication was an essential aspect of Methodism. The phenomenon to be observed was the central factor that could either be understood with the senses or with the help of instruments. The Methodists had a differentiated view of commonality, with conditions being either constricted, relaxed or a mixture of both. Phenomenon and commonality pointed the way to the indication, which was the third key concept in their system. In allocating the phenomena to commonalities they introduced a classification of sorts from which indications were derived. The concept of illness is decisive for the therapy. It is defined by a name, a description, an afflicted part of the body, and the treatment. The Methodist system is in principle holistic and assumes that any distinctive condition always involves the whole body. The *Methodists* were scathingly attacked for their views by physicians from Celsus (pr. 62–73) to Galen. The earliest followers of this tradition were the two *peregrini*, Thessalus of Tralles and Themison of Laodiceia in Syria (PLIN. nat. 25.80; 29.6; 29.9 and HANSON 1997: 298 f.), both outstanding physicians of their time: Thessalus, who was a leading physician in Rome under Nero, had a great numbers of pupils. Themison was a pupil of Asclepiades of Bithynia who went on to become an eminent practitioner in his own right (SCH. IUV. 10.221).

As well as the three traditions described by Celsus (Dogmatists, Empiricists, and Methodists) there was the Pneumatic tradition, which goes back to Agathinus of Sparta, a contemporary of the Emperor Nero (CIG 6292 and TIELMAN 2005). Agathinus was a pupil of Athenaeus of Attalia, who lived in

Pamphylia and was in contact with the Stoics. The Stoics attached special importance to the *pneuma* because it was for them the element from which the world fashioned the human body. Agathinus wrote a book in which he described the *pneuma* and came to the conclusion that it manifested in the pulse. However, the *Dogmatists*, the pupils of Herophilus and of Erasistratus, the *Empiricists*, and the *Methodists* had already pursued the same question so that it seems appropriate to question the independence of the Pneumatic tradition and assume that it was influenced by previously existent knowledge. It is a known fact that Agathinus was friendly toward the other traditions and one can therefore conclude that a lively exchange existed between them. Both the surgeon Leonidas of Alexandria, who inspired the surgeon and well-known writer Heliodorus, and Archigenes of Apamea, who is known to have been held in high esteem by Galen, were representatives of the Pneumatic tradition.

A fifth tradition existed in Alexandria in the second century BCE which, unlike the four groups described so far, was unknown and nameless. Research therefore refers to it as the *anonymous* tradition. It was ultimately Galen who was to blame for the fact that this tradition escaped scientific scrutiny for so long, because he omitted to mention it in his history (GRMEK/GOUREVITCH 1988). Danielle GOUREVITCH (1996: 129–132) provided evidence that, thanks to Marinus, his pupil Quintus and Quintus' pupil Numisianus, medicine flourished in Pergamum, Corinth, Rome, and Macedonia. These three physicians managed to extend humoral pathology by a localized concept of illness, an endeavor in which they were supported by anatomical, physiological, and pharmacological research on the one hand, and by clinical experience on the other. They were not as much concerned with excluding the one or other approach as with conducting a balanced study of the individual components that led to a concept made up of Hippocratic theories, discoveries made on the human body, and clinical method or experience.

II.4 – Medicine outside the traditions

Beside the medical traditions there were individual physicians who practiced medicine but did not belong to any of the groups mentioned. They can be divided into a group known from their writings – it is not necessary to establish in each case whether or not they were practicing medicine – and a group of definite practitioners. The sparse information we have on the latter group is epigraphic. The physicians who were also writers but did not belong to a particular group included, apart from their most prominent representative, Galen of Pergamum, also Aretaeus of Cappadocia, Scribonius Largus,

Pedanius Dioscorides of Anazarbus, Rufus of Ephesus, and Aulus Cornelius Celsus – who may have practiced medicine or just compiled medical knowledge (SCHULZE 1999).

Aretaeus of Cappacocia was a Greek physician who flourished in the middle of the first century CE and who drew on parts of the Pneumatic tradition (OBERHELMAN 1997 and KUDLIEN 1967: 100–106). His writings reveal marked interdependencies, in style as well as content, with the Hippocratic Corpus (Grmek 2000). Aretaeus describes every illness in precise terms, including its location, designation, and symptoms, as well as external circumstances, such as the time of year, for instance. The therapies he suggests include diets, bloodletting, and cupping. One of his contemporaries was Scribonius Largus, who left behind a collection of prescriptions entitled *Compositiones* (MEISSNER 1999: 198–201, SCONOCCHIA 1994, and DEICHGRÄBER 1950). Via his friends and colleagues Scribonius had political influence on the emperors Caligula and Claudius. He accompanied the latter as a military physician on the British campaign of 43 CE. His work contains a popular-scientific collection of pharmacological instructions for self-medication.

Pedanius Dioscorides of Anazarbus served temporarily as a military surgeon under Nero (MEISSNER 1999: 205 f. and RIDDLE 1994/1985). He produced a Materia Medica for colleagues in his field of work (DIOSC. De mat. med. I pr. 4) which differs from similar works by his predecessors, firstly, because he had practical experience of medicinal plants and, secondly, because it is not only an encyclopedia but a systematic introduction which places particular emphasis on pharmacological considerations. Dioscorides wrote not only for physicians but – like Scribonius Largus before him – also for their patients. His goal in doing so is twofold: to compose a new pharmacological standard work for his colleagues and to convey to lay-persons the specialist knowledge they needed to choose the right kind physician for themselves.

Rufus of Ephesus was a contemporary of Trajan who, during the Flavian dynasty, worked as a *peregrinus* in Egypt and Rome. Apart from Galen, he is the best known Greek physician of the second century CE in the Roman Empire. His encyclopedic work describes the principles of Hippocratic medicine but also presents justified reasons for distancing itself from it. He suggested that medical specialization led to superior methods that allowed medical knowledge and therapies to be targeted more directly at the individual patient than had been possible before. In his deliberations he distanced himself not only from the old traditions but also from his fellow practitioners. His writings were clearly the expression of a conflict with his medical rivals, from which he emerged as a successful imperial physician (MEISSNER 1999: 222). His influence lasted well into the Middle Ages.

CHRISTIAN SCHULZE proposes that Aulus Cornelius Celsus belongs to the ranks of writing physicians alongside Aretaeus of Cappadocia, Scribonius Largus, Pedanius Dioscorides of Anazarbus, and Rufus of Ephesus (SCHULZE 1999 and MUDRY 1994a/b). Celsus composed an encyclopedia of practical sciences. Of his contemplations, including those on agriculture, military matters, rhetoric, and law, only those on medicine have been preserved. Celsus' *De medicina libri octo* are invaluable testimonies of the cultural transfer of Greek medicine to the Roman Empire, particularly when it comes to questions of social history. It is not at all true that Celsus' work constitutes an inferior version of Greek developments (SELINGER 1999: 26). However, his efforts to develop his own specialist language are less convincing, particularly since his translations are full of errors. WELLMANN (1900) dubbed Celsus the Cicero of medical writers because he made medicine popular in the way Cicero did philosophy. Celsus introduced a nomenclature that would determine medicine for 1500 years. Another physician-author who did not belong to a group was Galen of Pergamum who is famous for his extensive writings. MATTERN (2013) presented her recent biography of Galen on the basis of the plentiful insights into his personal life she had garnered from these writings. Galen was born in 129 CE, during the reign of Hadrian, at Pergamum, one of the great sanctuaries dedicated to Asclepius. He died in Asia between 210 and 216 CE (NUTTON 1995a). At the age of 17, Galen began his studies of medicine and philosophy at Pergamum, before setting off for further learning to Smyrna, Corinth, and then Alexandria. After finishing his studies he first went back to Rome where he benefited, along with many others, from the desire of educated Romans to learn about Greek culture: the influx of scholars from the east was greatly promoted in the second century CE (GRUEN 1993: 223–225). Galen then travelled again (JONES 2012), arriving in Pergamum in 157 CE, where for some years he practiced successfully as a physician to gladiators (SCARBOROUGH 1971, and on gladiators in general ROBERT 1940). The gladiators were of high material value and received excellent medical care (MANN 2011: 104, WIEDEMANN 1995: 117, and NUTTON 1973: 163). While working as a physician to gladiators at Pergamum, Galen was able to enlarge the medical knowledge he already had by working with patients on a daily basis. Attending to the gladiators' wounds literally opened up new insights to him and helped him develop new methods. By verifying his theoretical knowledge empirically Galen was at the same time able to enhance his medical knowledge through practical application.

His treatment of gladiators formed the foundation of this professional development.

It was due to local political difficulties that Galen decided to go back to Rome in 162 CE, intending not to return to Pergamum until the 'stasis', or civil conflict, there abated (GAL. De praecogn. 14.622 K., SCHLANGE-SCHÖNINGEN 2003: 133 and NUTTON 1973: 164 f.). Four years later he left Rome again, this time because of the outbreak of the "Antonine Plague" (KOLLESCH 1981/1965), which was probably not a measles pandemic (MANLEY 2014) but smallpox that had spread across the entire Roman Empire (MATTERN 2013: 199–204 and NUTTON 2004: 24). From 169 CE, Galen remained in Rome, practicing in the imperial service, where emperors and courtiers were among his clientele. Many of his writings go back to that period: CARL GOTTLOB KÜHN's edition of his works comprises more than twenty volumes with over 20,000 pages of text – and that despite the fact that Galen's library was consumed by flames (BRODERSEN 2015). The goal of his materia medica, which adds to the works of previous authors the experience and insights he accumulated during his travels, was not only to compile but to extend, systemize and deepen the body of knowledge available (TOUWAIDE 1997 and HARIG 1974).

Galen belonged to no philosophical or medical traditions. In his view the *Corpus Hippocraticum* was more important than the teachings of the Methodists or Empiricists. He accused the Methodists of misunderstanding the principle of technical method. They ignored the value of practice, misinterpreted experience, and neglected medical theory (GAL. De meth. med. 10.126 f. K.). Of the Empiricists he was critical because they did not value observation highly enough. The superficial inspection of an occasional wound counted more to them than thorough practical training in anatomy (GAL. De anat. admin. 2.289 f. K.). Like the adherents of the anonymous tradition, Galen deepened his knowledge by applying the ideas of humoral pathology. Progress, he thought, was only possible if the Hippocratic considerations were heeded (GAL. De fac. nat. 2.44–47 K.). It was Galen's adherence to the Hippocratic tradition that helped him to be widely received and he, in turn, helped the Hippocratic tradition to be more widely received. Galen overcame the conservative influence of the Alexandrian anatomical literature by emphasizing the relevance of practice in his writings (GAL. De anat. admin. 2.283–289 K.). Moreover, by making every effort to convey his knowledge in lectures to the public (VON STADEN 1995), he contributed to the general medical education of society which, in quality as well as quantity, achieved a very high standard during the High Empire. Drawing upon a theory of causality, Galen explained illness as a shift in balance (GAL. Ars med. 1.314 f. K.).

The highest principle of therapy for Galen is prevention and his guidelines are consequently based on a healthy lifestyle. Dietetics and physical exercise come before medication and invasive surgery. He represents a medicine of his own, which is holistic and therefore also has scope for divine afflatus. For him, Asclepius was, next to Hippocrates, the embodiment of a good physician, because good medicine had to be ethical (GAL. In Hipp. Jusj. Comment. and ROSENTHAL 1956). This approach secured Galen high repute as a practitioner and as a theoretician. Throughout his life he was acknowledged in all strata of society. In his work *Deipnosophistae*, Athenaeus of Naucratis confirmed Galen's great importance during his own lifetime, pointing out that Galen composed more philosophical and medical books than all his predecessors put together (ATHEN. 1.1e; 26c–27d, and 3.115c–116a).

Galen conveyed Hellenic medicine and promoted its transfer to the Roman Empire. As part of the Muslim conquest of the ancient Mediterranean world, originally Hellenic medicine was transferred, mostly through the work of Avicenna, to the Arabic-Islamic Middle Ages. No new or independent scientific medical influences emerged during the period (WEISSER 1983) that saw mostly the absorption of ancient knowledge and thinking. Unsurprisingly therefore Avicenna is no more original compared to Galen than Galen is compared to the Hippocratic Corpus, seeing that the original Hellenic medical knowledge arrived in Europe via the Arabic-Islamic culture. It was the humanist bias towards Greece as well as the long overdue substitution of systematic manuals of the kind Avicenna also presented that facilitated Galen's renewed rise to prominence (STROHMAIER 1999: 109–111, 114–116, 125–127). His medical system formed the foundation of medicine right into the modern period (WITTERN 1999: 550). *Anathomia*, the major work published by Mondino de' Liuzzi (circa 1275–1326) in 1316, is the first post-ancient opus on human anatomy which, however, introduces fallacies arising from mistranslations of Galen's work. The 'unadulterated Galen' only came to be investigated in the mid-sixteenth century CE by pre-Vesalian anatomy. Because of the flaws of Galenian anatomy, Andreas Vesalius (1514–1564) asked for a new doctrine, which eventually rang in the end of Galen's predominance in the seventeenth century (WITTERN 1999: 567–571).

II.5 – Medical Practice

Illness and health are social and cultural constructs. Human beings continue to define their relationship with themselves and their bodies in interaction with the external factors that determine them. Health and illness, and the approaches to health and illness, must always be seen (as cultural history does) in the context of the cultural influences surrounding them (JÜTTE 1991). The imperial healing and health market was not restricted to physicians who benefited from and drew on the scientific medicine transferred from Greece. On this market services, other than self-treatment, were on offer that reflected the contemporary understanding of health and sickness and that covered everything from magic-demonic approaches to theurgic healing to rational-scientific medicine. They included sorcerers and miracle healers, healing cults, non-medical practitioners such as midwives, nurses and drug-dealers, and physicians (KORPELA 1987: 7; 16 and FISCHER 1979: 314.). Lay-treatment was traditionally performed by the *pater familias* (PLIN. nat. 25, 9 f., JACKSON 1988: 10 f., SCARBOROUGH 1969: 15–22, and ALBUTT 1921: 20–24) whose duties, even in the early period of the Roman Empire, included the provision of healthcare. He was expected to look after his own health and that of his family, slaves and cattle (COLUM. De re rustica 11.1.18). The various groups mentioned were not separate from each other but connected by their common concern, that of healing the sick. Their complex interaction could be informed by anything from friendliness to opposition (NUTTON 1995b: 4). A history of healers looks at the socio-historical context in more detail and depth than a history of physicians does. In later periods, say the Middle Ages or early modern times, research has tended to focus on the physician's perspective, demarcating it from the "lower-ranked healers" (JÜTTE 1994: 89 f.). Because of the latter group's inferior standing in society, it is rarely the object of historical research. And yet, a more comprehensive history of the healers, which includes social, economic, and cultural aspects, can make an important contribution to the history of civilization.

The assignation of the term *medicus* in Latin and ἰατρός / ἰατήρ in Greek to the practitioner of the medical profession and the related context of meaning pose certain questions. The meaning of the modern German word for physician (*"Arzt"*), for instance, differs considerably from that of the *medicus* or ἰατρός / ἰατήρ (CORDES 1994) in antiquity. While the etymology of the noun *medicus* is not helpful, the root of its Greek equivalent is more instructive: the terms ἰατρός / ἰατήρ derive from the verb ἰάομαι (to heal), which has the Indo-European root *isa-io. The Indo-European root *isnió, to which the verb ἰαίνω (to refresh or quicken) traces back is also relevant. RECHENAUER (2000: 386 footnote 3) refers to a Linear-B-tablet from Pylos that already mentioned an *i-a-te* (singular noun iater, Py Eq 146 and VENTRIS 1973:547).

The German word *Arzt*, on the other hand, goes back to the epithet used for public physicians in antiquity, which from Hellenic times had been ἀρχιατρός and which became *archiater* in late Latin. While the terms ἰατρός / ἰατήρ focus on the activity of healing, the German word *Arzt* – in the sense of ἀρχιατρός – emphasizes the physician's official and social status. The meaning of the ancient terms ἰατρός / ἰατήρ consequently covers a much wider range than the connotations of *Arzt* seem to suggest at first glance. The Greek terms are more about the patient and the act of care-giving and therefore better suited to describe the great diversity of healer groups which are all connected by their healing activities (MEISSNER 1997 and KOLLESCH 1979: 508).

Aside from the masculine form *medicus* or ἰατρός / ἰατήρ one also finds the feminine equivalents, *medica* or ἰατρίνη, but their meaning has remained unclear and is the subject of controversy in research (KISLINGER 2005, SCHU-MACHER 2001: 217 f., and SCHUBERT/HUTTNER 1999: 488). The case of a woman called Phanostrate, who lived in the first half of the fourth century BCE, can illuminate this problem. The inscription on Phanostrate's gravestone refers to her as a physician (ἰατρίνη) and a midwife (μαῖα, IG II/III² 6873). The stone depicts four children and a woman whose hand Phanostrate is shaking. The picture may contain a reference to her profession (POMEROY 1997: 133). The dual designation was initially thought to signify that midwives were only concerned with childbirth, while the physicians' field of activity was much wider. The use of the term ἰατρίνη or *medica* is therefore ambivalent because it could mean, on the one hand, that her scope of duties went beyond that of a midwife (ἰατρόμαια / μαῖα / obstetrix). On the other hand, the term ἰατρίνη / medica may have been used synonymously with ἰατρόμαια / μαῖα / obste-trix, which would mean that both terms cover the same field of activity. This would explain why in later times a medically trained midwife was referred to as ἰατρόμαια, a synthesis of ἰατρός and μαῖα. (GUMMERUS 1932: 15 and BAADER 1967: 233).

In his work *Politics* Aristotle distinguished between practitioners (δημι-ουργός) and scientifically educated physicians (ἀρχιτεκτονικός), setting both apart from medically educated lay-healers (πεπαιδευμένος περὶ τὴν τέχνην, ARISTOT. pol. 3.11: 1282 a 3 f. and GAL. De libr. propr. 19.9 K.). Anyone could become a physician by seeking instruction in τέχνη ἰατρική from a practicing physician, as stipulated by the Hippocratic Oath (HIPPOKR. Jusj. II).

καὶ διδάξειν τὴν τέχνην ταύτην, ἢν χρηίζωσι μανθάνειν, ἄνευ μισθοῦ καὶ ξυγγραφῆς, παραγγελίης τε καὶ ἀκροήσιος καὶ τῆς λοιπῆς ἁπάσης μαθήσιος μετάδοσιν ποιήσασθαι υἱοῖσί τε ἐμοῖσι καὶ τοῖσι τοῦ ἐμὲ διδάξαντος καὶ μαθηταῖσι συγγεγραμμένοις τε καὶ ὡρκισμένοις νόμῳ ἰητρικῷ, ἄλλῳ δὲ οὐδενί.

To teach them this art, if they are willing to learn it, without fee or indenture; to impart precept, oral instruction, and all other instruction to my own sons, the sons of my teacher, and to indentured pupils who have taken the physician's oath, but to nobody else.

It was the declared goal of this τέχνη to preserve health as a highest good by applying prophylactic or restorative measures. The oath regulated the medical training by giving it a contractual foundation that amounted to a professional-ethical pledge: a student is admitted for training by a teacher who is an expert in the art of medicine (SCHUBERT 2005: 20 f.). The student will only receive lessons if he vows to adhere to particular medical standards of behavior. This is about the ethics of medical experts in relation to those who need healing and those who are willing to heal (CAVANAUGH 2017). Once the oath has been taken by the student, the teacher begins to instruct and lecture him on general medical rules, bedside behavior and consultation. In return, the pupil promises to support his teacher in times of need and in his old age, and to pass on his art to his own sons. Professional competence becomes part of a family structure. The sons of the teacher also became physicians and did this willingly because of the status it would give them. These ideas are projected onto the figure of Hippocrates in a concentrated form, for instance when PHERECYDES (FGrHist 3 F 59) declares him to have descended from a family of physicians that goes back seven generations or in the claim that he was a direct descendent of Asclepius in the 25th generation of physicians (SCHUBERT 2005: 61–66).

The students acquired empirical knowledge by receiving practical bedside tuition and participating in consultations. Healthcare was not usually provided in a clinical context but by physicians visiting their patients at home or by patients attending the *iatreion* or the *tabernae medicae* or *medicinae* in order to consult a physician (HARIG 1971: 182–187). The only established forms of clinical care were the *valetudinaria* where soldiers and slaves were admitted and cared for because their superiors were keen to keep them fit for working and fighting (WILMANNS 1995: 103–116, 136–138 and HARIG 1971: 188–195).

Efforts to introduce regulations in the Roman Empire were initially restricted to the guaranteed provision of medical care. In order to achieve this, Iulius Caesar granted Roman citizenship, in 46 BCE, to foreign physicians practicing in Rome and made sure that medical provision was available to the troops (SUET. Iul. 42.1 and DIOD. 53.30). Also at that time the Ephesian physicians were granted exemption from tax (KNIBBE 1981/1982 and WILMANNS 1995: 66). Regulations that promoted institutionalization are mostly known from the imperial period: Augustus freed the physicians from civil obligations and tax liability by granting them immunity (CASS. DIO 53.30.3.). Vespasian confirmed this decree and, in 74 CE, introduced the right to professional representation (FISCHER 1979). Professional associations were formed to represent the interests of physicians and organize specialized professional development (BELOW 1953: 30 f.). Tax exemption, or *immunitas,* was confirmed by Hadrian in 117 CE. Antoninus Pius restricted immunity to the official town physicians, who from then on also had to be appointed by the authorities (DIG. 27.1.6.2 f.). Depending on the size of a commune, immunity would not be granted to more than five, seven, or ten physicians. Institutionalized medical training was promoted by Severus Alexander, who granted state funding to certain physicians to enable them to teach, and he made public lecture halls available to them (BELOW 1953: 43). Emperor Constantine granted all physicians freedom from military service and taxation, a decree that was reintroduced by Julian in 362 CE. What was not achieved by the end of the ancient period was to make theoretical and practical training compulsory for all physicians. This was certainly due in part to the fact that medical theories were based on philosophy rather than natural science (SCHUMACHER 1963), which was also why the premises from which their theories derived were rather prone to speculation and interpretation.

A particular situation arose under the Flavians, when physicians were occasionally placed at the service of the general public. Slave doctors now practiced within the *familia Caesaris* or in private households (SCHUMACHER 2001: 215), as is apparent from the large family graves where the un-free physicians were also buried. While these slave doctors were usually poor, they had the possibility to gain freedom or social advancement in recognition of their medical services. Inscriptions found in eastern Greece and Rome from the second century CE onward prove that the title ἀρχιατρός was assigned to public physicians (KUDLIEN 1985: 42 ff.). As ἀρχιατρός, such a physician became a public office holder. The long-term result of this development was the emergence of a privileged class of imperial physicians whose office became hereditary (CIG 2987 and SEG 17.527).

While restrictions applied to the number of public physicians, the number of private physicians practicing alongside them was unlimited. Their social status was similar to that of craftspeople. The physicians, who were employed in the service of the imperial family or the senators, had a good reputation and income and led comfortable lives. The two Stertinii brothers, both official physicians to the emperor, were among the wealthiest families (KRUG 1993: 208–212). The first private physicians were Greeks, slaves, and freedmen

(SCHUMACHER 2001: 215 f.). With the beginning of the imperial period they were first joined by large numbers of un-free practitioners, mostly hailing from Greece and Asia Minor (JACKSON 1988: 56 and KORPELA 1987: 53 f.), and only over time by freeborn Romans (KUDLIEN 1986: 20 ff.).

The practicing physicians had to earn a good name for themselves in public, overcome the mistrust they encountered and prove their skills to the lay-people (SELINGER 1999: 29). The art of a physician therefore depended on the judgment of the lay-population rather than on scientific criteria. Physicians had to face the vibrant healer and health market, awaken medical sensitivity, explain complex pathophysiological aspects to laymen, and impart on them the understanding that biological systems were dynamic and largely unpredictable. In addition to all that they also had to compete with their colleagues, a fact that explains why the first ten chapters of the Hippocratic volume on diseases constitute an instruction on medical debate (HIPPOKR. Morb. I and WITTERN 1998b: 34–37). This seems to indicate that there was much competition among the physicians and that they were under great pressure to prove themselves to the public, even in the very early days of medical practice.

A third group aside from the public and private practitioners were the military physicians, who worked alongside the paramedics and veterinary surgeons to provide medical services (WESCH-KLEIN 1998: 71–90 and WILMANNS 1995). Evidence of an organized medical service in the military is available onwards from the time of Augustus, when fundamentally new conditions were established. Before then, the troops used to be based close to cities and rural settlements so that they could be tended to by civilian physicians. Now the Empire's expansionist policy made it necessary for medical care to be available to the troops in the remote garrisons. Some emperors continued to travel with their own physicians, such as Tiberius for instance (VELL. 2.114.2), or Claudius, who was accompanied on his British campaign by the physician Stertinius Xenophon from Cos. During the Dacian Wars, Trajan was looked after by Criton, and, in the fourth century CE, the Emperor Julian took his physician Oribasius along on his campaigns (WESCH-KLEIN 1998: 76).

Military physicians practiced in the sickrooms or in the *valetudinaria* (RISSE 1999: 38–56). The first *valetudinaria* are documented for the northern army as early as around the birth of Christ (KÜNZL 1991). The conquest of Germania meant that the soldiers needed medical care in a territory with unfavorable climatic conditions and without the necessary infrastructure. The reason for setting up these *valetudinaria* was to ensure that fully fit soldiers were available locally and that competent medical help was on hand. Each legion had a separate building to house its sick, just like the big military *castra*. No such establishments were available to the naval forces or to the urban Roman *vigils,* however. There is no evidence of *valetudinaria* in the camps of late antiquity, probably because the greater mobility of the armies at that time rendered them obsolete. As during the Republic, the sick were left behind in families, either in the city or in the country, where they were cared for (WESCH-KLEIN 1998: 78). Some of the patients were taken in by the Christian *xenodochia* provided by the church.

Military physicians provided medical care to the troops (SAMAMA 2017 and BREITWIESER/ HUMER/POLLHAMMER/ARNOTT 2018). Their tasks included the application of fast-working therapeutic measures in acute situations, as well as the subsequent provision of curative and follow-up care. To aid recuperation, soldiers were sometimes sent to therapeutic baths. During a war, the physicians were mostly occupied with wound care or surgery (JACKSON 1988: 112–137). Physicians in charge of wound treatment in the army were called *medicus,* as were soldiers who acted as barber-surgeons (*miles medicus*) in the army (ISRAELOWICH 2016 and SCARBOROUGH 1969: 66–75). One of the two sons of Asclepius – Machaon – is the classic embodiment of the Homeric physician, since he was already described as a barber surgeon (SCH. HOM. Il. 15.515 and STEGER 2000: 32).

There is, rather surprisingly, no separate recent literature on military medicine in Antiquity except SAMAMA (2017) for Greece and BREITWIESER/ HUMER/ POLLHAMMER/ARNOTT (2018) for Rome. No war surgery as such was developed and the wounded soldiers were treated by general surgeons. Celsus mentions the treatment of wounds, bleeding, and inflammation, the extraction of foreign objects and bullets, and the amputation of limbs (CELS. art. 5.26.21–24; 7.5.1–5 and 7.33.1–2). Specialists were at hand in some places, even for animals (*medici veterinarii*). Among the latter, mule doctors (*mulomedici*), cattle doctors (*pecuarii*), and horse doctors (*equarii*) were prominent (LORENZ 2000: 190 f.).

BLIQUEZ (2015) gives a comprehensive and up to date overview of surgical instruments in Greek and Roman times. He both presents archaeological findings and testimonies from the literary sources. Somewhat misleading is the title of his book, "Tools of Asclepius". The question as to whether surgical interventions took place in the Asclepieia is discussed controversially by research (III.5.1).

In performing their duties physicians not only helped the sick and wounded. Their surgical interventions also allowed them to study the human body in-depth and to refine the anatomical knowledge they had acquired mostly by dissecting animals (SELINGER 1999: 30 f.). As well as injured soldiers, wounded gladiators or travelers who had been hurt by robbers were also welcome study objects for the physicians (CELS. pr. 43). And lastly, physicians were able to widen their specialist knowledge by studying new healing methods when their work took them to foreign parts of the Roman Empire (WESCH-KLEIN 1998: 50).

There were other groups apart from the physicians that were active on the healing and health market. It is difficult to draw a clear line between them and the physicians in individual cases: among them were masseurs, nurses, and manufacturers or dealers of drugs and medicines. In his history of medicine Pliny (29.1–27) also mentioned the ἰατραλειπτική introduced by Herodicus of Selymbria (PLIN. nat. 29.4 and 4.47), an art in which gymnastics played a prominent part. Herodicus thought that illness arose from misguided lifestyles and he therefore recommended treatments such as sweat baths, rubbing down, and gymnastics. When Pliny the Younger fell ill in 97 CE he was successfully treated by the Egyptian freedman Harpocras. He expressed his gratitude to Harpocras by gaining Egyptian and Roman citizenship for him. By using salves, oils, alternating baths, and diets Harpocras was able to save Pliny from even worse afflictions. SCHUMACHER's characterization of the ἰατραλείπτης as a homeopath (2001: 217) is questionable because he is confusing naturopathic and homeopathic concepts.

The second group of non-physicians are the nurses (capsarii / ὑπηρέτεις). They are difficult to identify because the term capsarius / ὑπηρέτης often designates a particular kind of servant (SCHUMACHER 2001: 215). The same problems apply to both nouns. One can cautiously assume that the ὑπηρέτεις were assistants who mixed ointments and applied bandages or splints. The contribution made to the healing process by the capsarius / ὑπηρέτης remains unclear. Capsarii are known to have provided nursing services in the Roman army (GUMMERUS 1932: 14). In ambulant care they could also undergo further training and become medici (WILMANNS 1995: 118 f.).

Finally, there are the producers and dealers of drugs and medicines who also belonged to the group of non-physicians. They were called by a variety of names, including aromatarii, myropolae, pharmacopolae, pigmentarii, seplasiarii, thuriarii, and unguentarii (TOTELIN 2016). Because they not only supplied clients with their products but also advised them, they were important contributors to the healing and health market, particularly because they needed to be able to analyze what their clients suffered from before they could advise them. What remains unclear in the individual cases is which herbs they sold and how extensive their medical tasks were (KORPELA 1987: 21). There is evidence that the φαρμακοπώλαι not only sold medicines but also treated illnesses (DIOD.

32.11.2.). Some also sold cosmetic substances (OV. ars 2.489. Petron. 102.5; 126.2 and MART. 3.3.1). The fact that they were attacked by the physicians (GAL. De fasc. 43A, 770 K.) seems to imply that they were seen as rivals because they were consulted by the patients. On the other hand, there is also documentary evidence of the two groups working together (SCRIB. LARG. comp. 122).

III

The Practice of Asclepius

III.1 – The myth of Asclepius and his healing cult

The curing of illnesses was a task that fell to any deity or hero who had the superhuman powers to achieve such a feat, but the healing cult centres on a few representatives only (CROON 1986 and JAYNE 1925), of whom Apollo is one. In the Iliad he is said to have sent the plague by the shooting of an arrow, but also to have lifted the epidemic once reconciliation had taken place (KRUG 1993: 149 and KÖRNER 1929: 36–38). Anatomical votives reveal the deities which were revered for their healing powers: they include Heracles in his role as a protector and healer, the oriental Zeus of the imperial period, also female deities of birth and childcare, such as Demeter and Kore, Eileithyia and Artemis, Minerva and Juno, as well as Carmenta, the goddess of childbirth and springs. The votive offerings presented to these deities of childbirth were mostly depictions of human body parts such as female breasts and sexual organs (FORSÈN 1996: 134–144). The dedicatory inscriptions on these relief votives tend to provide little evidence other than these references to limbs and to the names of the supplicant and of the deity to which the offering was made (FORSÈN 1996: 133–159, COMELLA 1986/1981 and TABANELLI 1962). What they do reveal is information regarding the dominant pathology, because they depict the diseased body parts which had either been healed or commended to the protection of a particular deity (TURFA 1994). Demeter and her daughter Kore were revered as a unity (FORSÈN 1996: 142–144). According to the myth, Asclepius hid Heracles in the Spartan sanctuary of the Eleusinian Demeter in order to heal his injuries (PAUS. 20.5). HUPFLOHER (2000: 56 f. with IG 623), on the other hand, goes too far in my view when she describes the Eleusinian sanctuary as a health centre. Eleithyia was *the* goddess of childbirth par excellence, but she was also worshipped because she looked after older children and because she possessed healing powers (FORSÈN 1996: 135).

Among the local heroes was also Amynus, worshipped since the sixth century BCE as a healing hero and, later, as a god in his own sanctuary on the southern slope of the Areopagus in Athens (FORSÈN 1996: 146). Amynus warded off evil and protected human beings from illness. Countless votive reliefs have been discovered in the Amyneion, which provide evidence not only

of an Amynus cult but also of cults to Asclepius and Hygieia (KRUG 1993: 148).
In Eleusis a certain Oresinius was revered, and in Marathon and Rhamnous
a hero called Aristomachus (ANECD. BEKK. I 262.16 and 263.11). Behind both
names the hero Iatros is concealed, who was often referred to by his title alone
(GRAF 1998: 245, PARKER 1997: 176 f. and SCHNALKE 1990: 9 f.). Amphiaraus
of Boeotia, who was worshipped as a god in Rhamnous and Oropus, was also
one of the healing heroes, but no offerings of body parts were made to him
(KRUG 1993: 153–155). He could bring healing to the sick in their dreams and
he also had a small sanctuary close to the Hephaisteion in Athens.

Apollo Medicus was very popular in Rome from 433 BCE at the latest,
and the goddesses Ceres and Diana arrived in Rome from Sicily via Magna
Graecia (NUTTON 1999b: 1110 f.). Of all the healing cults which were scattered across Rome and its growing empire, the cults of Asclepius, Heracles
and Serapis were the most prominent. Like Asclepius, Heracles belonged to a
younger generation of deities. Both were close to humans and both were able
to release humans from various kinds of evil: Asclepius cured illness and Heracles freed humans from monsters that plagued them. Lucian satirizes their
relationship in *Dialogs of the Gods* where he has Heracles complain to Zeus
about Asclepius being of superior rank (LUCIAN. dial. deor. 13). A joint festival, »Σωτηρία καὶ Ἡρακλεία«, introduced to Pergamum during the reign of
Eumenes II. (197–159 BCE), is proof of the cult (SCHEER 1993: 141 f.). This is
known from an inscription at the Asclepieion (AvP VII.3 No. 3): Prince Athenaeus, the younger brother of Eumenes II and Attalos II, was honoured at that
festival by being appointed Agonothetes. Ἡρακλεία is a festival in honor of
Heracles and Σωτηρία is celebrated in honor of Asclepius. Σωτήρ was a name
commonly used for Asclepius at Pergamum (OHLEMUTZ 1940: 156).

For the Greeks, Heracles was the archetypal hero (his Roman name is
Hercules): a human being who achieved immortality through his deeds and
who was worshipped widely (FORSÈN 1996: 149 f. and BURKERT 1979: 78–98).
Whether it was in a Herculean temple in the Boeotian village of Hyettus, in
Messene on Sicily, or at Geronthrae in Laconia – the sick could come to any
of these places to be healed by Heracles. Heracles was also worshipped in the
thermal springs of Aidepsos on Euboia (STRAB. 9.4.13).

To Serapis, a new deity of the early Ptolemaic period, a place was allocated next to the famous and highly respected Isis. The cult of Isis is one of
the mystery religions that were among the most vibrant manifestations of the
religious life in the imperial period (MERKELBACH 2001, CHRIST 1995: 568 ff.,
and VIDMAN 1970). It reflects the religious, cultural, and political synthesis of
Egyptian and Greek traditions. Serapis combines within himself the Egyptian

gods Osiris, Apis, Amun, and Re, and was seen as identical with the most sublime beings of other religions, such as Zeus, for instance. The new Serapis cult absorbed the Greek tradition of Eleusis by equating Isis with Demeter, and the tradition of the Bacchic mysteries by equating Osiris, Serapis, and Dionysus, and it links these with the Egyptian myths and rituals. The establishment of the Isis and Serapis mysteries in the whole eastern Mediterranean region was facilitated by the cultural policy of the first two Ptolemaic kings and can be seen as one of the most momentous results of the meeting of Greek and Egyptian cultures (ASSMANN 2000).

The main reasons why Asclepius occupied such an eminent place among the healing deities were firstly that his healing cult formed the core of a religious medicine in the occident (SCHNALKE 1990: 7 f.) and, secondly, that his healing cult contributed considerably to the provision of healthcare in ancient times. While there is scholarly consensus now regarding the cultic aspect of religious medicine, the medical practice which formed part of the healing cults has so far not been fully acknowledged by research. It is noticeable in this context that the treatments carried out in the healing cults often involved illnesses that were not (or no longer) accessible to the commonly used medical methods described in the specialist literature of the time (GRAF 1998: 243 f.).

The significance of the healing cult is – as FRITZ GRAF points out correctly – intimately linked to the myth, and every sanctuary is a focal point for myths and rituals (GRAF 1992b: 159 and, in more general terms, BURKERT 1972: 39–45). On his father's side, Asclepius descended from the Gods. He was elevated from hero to deity in the late sixth century BCE (HOM. Il. 2.731 f.; 4.194; 219. HES. Frg. 125, PIND. Pyth. 3.5 ff., EUR. Alc. 3 f., and 122 ff.). The myth speaks of his father, Apollo (Hom. Hymn. 16), who was worshipped as the sender and healer of illness. In the Iliad, Apollo sends a plague (λοιμός) with his arrows, but he also sends healing to the Greeks after they have placated him with ritual offerings (HOM. Il. 1.42–53; 314 f. and 467–474) in a great feast involving food, drink, dance and the singing of a paean. The cleansing was not so much an act of hygiene but rather a cultic washing away of a sacrilege (LEVEN 1997a: 17). On the other hand there is also evidence that the people of Rome were plagued by a cruel epidemic in 433 BCE and that they decided to build a temple for Apollo hoping that would induce him to free them from this evil (LIV. 4.25.3 f. and 4.29.7). In 431 BCE this temple was consecrated to Apollo on Campus Marius where Apollo Medicus was venerated (HAEHLING VON LANZENAUER 1996: 18 and BECHER 1970: 214–216).

Asclepius shared his mortality and death with other heroes (OV. fast. 6, 743 ff., DIOD. 4.71.1–4, KRUG 1993: 122, and VLASTOS 1948: 274); and it was only his heroization that gave rise to the healing cult (FARNELL 1921: 234–279) which then spread from Epidaurus across the Mediterranean world and even into the Gallic and German territories, reaching its acme in the fourth century BCE. The myth of Asclepius began with Homer, whose description of this myth also constituted the beginning of its processing. BLUMENBERG (1979/1971) demonstrated how reading a myth that has become part of a literary tradition initiates the process of its cultural-historical reception. In the processing of the myth he includes diachronic phenomena such as its reception, citation, and transformation, which he sees as belonging to the effective history of mythology. Variants of the myth were summarized by Diodorus in his late Hellenic synthesis (DIOD. 4.71.1–3 and STEGER 2000: 31–38). Diodorus' deliberations were based on the account of the mythographers: Asclepius was the son of Apollo and Coronis. He was born with special faculties and intelligence and was keen to study medicine because he wished to be able to help human beings. He discovered many remedies which were beneficial to human health. Among his outstanding gifts was the ability to cure even patients whose condition was considered hopeless. Because of the astonishing results he achieved he acquired the reputation of having the power to bring the dead back to life.

The response to Asclepius' skill was not only positive. Hades complained to Zeus that the number of dead had gone down considerably as a result of Asclepius' interference. Zeus found Asclepius guilty and, in his wrath, slayed him with a thunderbolt (cf. EUS. Pr. Ev. 2.2.34 and LUCIAN. Peregr. 4). Asclepius had broken the law by extending the life of his patients beyond the biological norm, a bold step, for which he had to pay with his life, but which also allowed him to work miracles in his sanctuaries later: he added an epiphanic component to his sphere of activities and distanced himself at the same time from the work of his son, Machaon, who symbolized the early Asclepius. HOMER (Il. 2.732) described Machaon as a barber surgeon, while Podalirius, Asclepius' second son, was allocated the sphere of internal medicine (CORDES 1991). Diodorus concludes his synthesis by proposing that Apollo had the Cyclopes killed out of revenge because they had fashioned the thunderbolts for Zeus. Zeus, in return, punished Apollo by forcing him to serve a human being. So much for the myth of Asclepius.

The propagation of the Asclepius cult started from Epidaurus, which is also the origin of the two iconographic types from the first half of the fourth century BCE: one is the bearded Asclepius who stands leaning on the snake-entwined rod (fig. 3). It was created around 380 BCE and is known as the Giustini type (MEYER 1994: 26 ff., MEYER 1988, and NEUGEBAUER 1921). In this pose Asclepius appears restful, exuding closeness and devotion to the

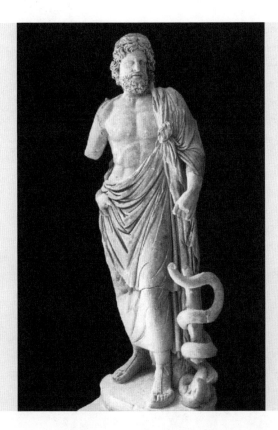

devotees. The other type is sitting down, with a serpent winding beneath his throne. This latter type traces back to the cultic image of the Epidaurian Asclepieion created by the sculptor Thrasymedes in 370 BCE (Athens, National Archaeological Museum 173, 1330, 1338, 1339).

PAUSANIAS (2.27.2) related that the cultic statue made of gold and ivory was half the size of that of the Olympian Zeus in Athens (reconstruction in IAKOVIDIS 1985: 131). The deity is depicted sitting on a throne grasping a staff in one hand and holding the other hand above the serpent's head. A dog is lying on the ground (LORENZ 2000: 211–214). On the throne the deeds of Argive heroes are depicted, such as the fight of Bellerophon with the chimera, or Perseus beheading the Gorgon Medusa. A copy of the same image appears on the back of the Epidaurian Drachma, which bears the laurel-crowned Apollo on the obverse (FRANKE 1969: 62 f. fig. 2). Both these attributes, serpent and staff, appear frequently as representations of the healing cult of Asclepius. In Greco-Roman times the snake winding around the staff was the symbol of Asclepius, the god of healing. It came into use again during the Renaissance (SCHOUTEN 1967) and over time, with its increasing detachment from Asclepius, became a universal symbol for medicine and pharmacy (figs. 1–10 in STEGER 2000: 21–25). As is apparent from the votive reliefs, another element, that of the temple sleep, was added to the serpent and the staff. These depictions of healings show Asclepius alone or surrounded by his family, but mostly with his daughter Hygieia, the embodiment of health. In Rome Asclepius is Latinized into Aesculapius, while Hygieia becomes Valetudo and later Salus (SOBEL 1990 and LORENZ 1988: 2f.). Aesculapius derives from the earlier *Aischklapios*, an old Epidaurian variant of the name. Two epigraphs from Tiber Island in Rome mention the old form *Aiscolapio* (CIL VI 4.4, 30482 and 30846). Aesculapius, as an Augustan deity, receives the attribute "Augustus" (AE 1993: 1221). The etymology of the name Asclepius remains unclear (KRUG 1993: 122 and STEGER 2005a: 15).

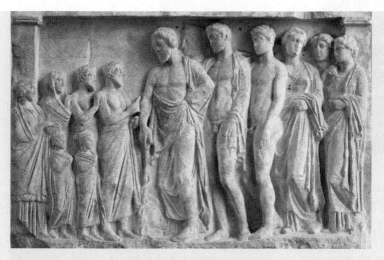

Fig. 4 – Votive relief: Asclepius and his family with devotees

A votive relief from the first half of the fourth century BCE (fig. 4) shows a group of mortals approaching a line of gods with their hands raised in reverence. A sacrificial pig crouches on the ground. Asclepius leads the group of gods on the right. He is depicted in the familiar manner, with beard, cloak and rod. He is followed by Hygieia, seen from the back, and his sons, Machaon and Podalirius. Asclepius' daughters Iaso, Aceso and Panacea are also part of the group, having been admitted to the family around the end of the fifth century BCE, once the situation had settled after the turmoil of the Peloponnesian War (BENEDUM 1990: 225). Hygieia, too, was not integrated into the family until later (STAFFORD 1998: 163–170, DE LUCA 1991, and SOBEL 1990), but, unlike Asclepius's spouse, Epione, she became closely attached to the realm of healing (PAUS. 2.4.5 and 2.27.6). The cult merely acknowledges Hygieia as the daughter of Asclepius, but she was in fact revered at almost the same level as her father. Many stone sculptures, including the important groups by Scopas of Paros in Gortyna (Arcadia) and Tegea, show her standing at her father's side (PAUS. 8.28.1 and 8.47.1). Asclepius is occasionally also assisted by servants of the sanctuary or relatives of the patient (LEY 1997 and HOLTZMANN 1984). These illustrations usually depict Asclepius standing by the patient's bedside. A votive relief from Athens shows Asclepius healing a woman (votive relief from Piraeus, Mus. Inv. No. 405 and KRUG 1993 fig. 57). Interestingly, no votive reliefs remain from Epidaurus which seems to indicate that scenes of this kind were recorded in some other medium there. In the second century BCE a child-like figure called Telesphorus was included at Pergamum (PAUS. 2.11.7). His name, which translates as "he who brings things to a good end", can be seen as the programme of Asclepian medicine. Telesphorus is often shown standing at the God's feet, as for instance in a late-Hellenistic Asclepius portrayal from Cos (fig. 5), or on a gem from the third century CE (Hanover, Kestner Museum No K 1674 and KRUG 1993: 125 Fig. 52b).

The child-like figure with its hooded cloak has something gnome-like about it. A small copper coin from the city of Synaus (Phrygia) from the third century CE bears the head of Asclepius on the front and a child clad in a cowl on the reverse. This is Telesphorus, who was companion and assistant to Asclepius (FRANKE 1969: 64 fig. 14). Serpent, rod, and temple sleep are typical attributes of a hero cult and have been testified for the cult of Asclepius from the fifth century BCE at the latest, in statues, figurines, votive reliefs, coins and gems, but not for the early Asclepius (BENEDUM 1990: 214).

The most important and famous sanctuary to Asclepius was situated in a high valley six miles south of the ancient city of Epidaurus (HENNING 1989, IAKOVIDIS 1985: 127–155, TOMLINSON 1983, CHARITONIDOU 1978, PAPACHATZIS 1978, and BURFORD 1969). The oldest remains date from the late sixth century BCE, which means that Epidaurus was probably the original site of Asclepius' worship (STEGER 2000: 33 f., BENEDUM 1996, and KRUG 1993: 128 f.). The poet Isyllus locates the birthplace of Asclepius there (IG IV² 1.128 and VLASTOS 1948: 275 f.). In 395 CE Epidaurus was raided by the Goths, and in 426 CE its history ended with Theodosius II closing down the pagan sanctuary. Between 1879 and 1928 the sanctuary was excavated by Panagiotis Kavadias. French archaeologists and the Greek Archaeological Service have been working there since 1948 (map in HART 2000: 56).

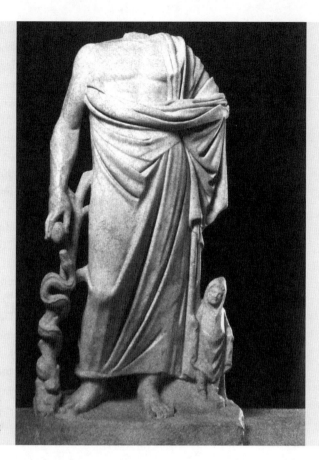

Fig. 5 – Asclepius
with Telesphorus
on his left

Apollo was worshipped in sanctuaries at Delphi, Delos, and Paros, and in each of them a separate sacred area was dedicated to Asclepius. At Epidaurus too, the mythical son of Apollo was able to build on the earlier tradition of the local deity Apollo Maleatas. Prehistoric finds from Mount Kynortion, one and half miles south-east of the Asclepieion, seem to point to the Maleatas having his own cultic precinct there (TOMLINSON 1983: 22 with footnotes 13 and 92–94).

We generally observe with the dissemination of the cult of Asclepius that – not only in Epidaurus, but also in Corinth and Cos – it was rooted in the preceding Apollo cult. By the second half of the fifth century BCE the veneration of Asclepius was sufficiently established for the cult to spread further afield from Epidaurus (LECOS/PENTOGALOS 1986 and TOMLINSON 1983). That most of the later founded Asclepieia have even until now not been investigated is due to the fact that hardly any of them have been excavated. RIETHMÜLLER (2005) and MELFI (2007) have assembled all the material that is available. We can say with some certainty that few sanctuaries grew to be as big and significant as Epidaurus and it can therefore be alleged that Epidaurus was the starting point of the cult and that it occupied an eminent position. When it comes to the architectural design of the later affiliations, the sanctuary on Cos soon became a model for others (COARELLI 1986: 7 f.). HART provides a good semi-quantitative overview (fig. 6) of the geographical dissemination and distribution of the Asclepian cult: Asclepian sanctuaries were founded in Delphi, Sicyon, Corinth and on the island of Aegina. The Asclepieion in Delphi has no temple complex. It was situated behind the Athenian Treasury below the temple terrace. The Apollonian cult was also prominent in Delphi, attracting devotees in large numbers (KRUG 1993: 156). In the course of the fifth century BCE it became possible for the Asclepius cult in Corinth to take over from the cult of Apollo (KRUG 1993: 142–145, LANG 1977, and WEGNER 1961: 979). Pausanias' description of Corinth is brief because not much was left of the city when he visited it after Lucius Mummius had ordered its destruction in 146 BCE (PAUS. 2.4.5). The sanctuary at Corinth was entirely destroyed in 396 CE during the invasion by the Visigoths under Alaric. There was an Asclepieion in Aegina, which was also frequented by Athenians (ARISTOPH. Vesp. 122 f.), but no archaeological evidence has been found for it so far.

In 420 BCE, with the help of Epidaurian delegates, the cult of Asclepius was transferred to Athens (IG IV² 41), where work was in progress to establish a sanctuary for Asclepius. The deity was first received into the Eleusinion until his own sanctuary was completed (SEG 25.226 and WICKKISER 2008: 62–72). It is possible that an Athenian attack took place on Epidaurus in 430 BCE with the aim of carrying Asclepius and his cult off to Athens (THUC. 2.56.4. PLUT. Per. 35, and MIKALSON 1984: 220). This kind of cultic transfer was driven by economic rather than political interests because an Asclepian sanctuary was seen as a good source of income (GARLAND 1992: 123 f.). Another reason was that, at the time, the citizens of Athens still had vivid memories of the devastating plague (λοιμός) and the impact it had on their lives (WICKKISER 2010). The epidemic broke out in the summer of 430 BCE (THUC. 2.47.2 f.) and raged on until the summer of 428 BCE (THUC. 3.87.1 f.), returning in the winter of 427/426 BCE for yet another year, until the winter of 426/425 BCE (MIKALSON 1984: 217 f.). In those five years it killed off a fourth to a third of the Athenian population (HORSTMANSHOFF 1992: 53 and LEVEN 1991).

In the contemporary medical jargon the term λοιμός designated a disease from which no one was safe (HIPPOKR. Flat. 6.97 L.). Details about the disease can only be derived from the ancient sources, for instance from Thucydides' account which consists mainly in a list of symptoms (THUC. 2.9 f.). Using the

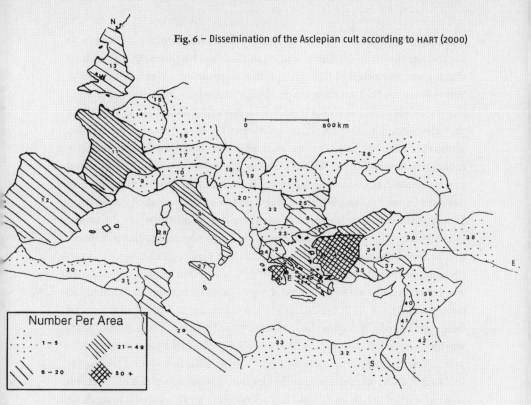

Fig. 6 – Dissemination of the Asclepian cult according to HART (2000)

Number Per Area

- ∴ 1 – 5
- ⫽ 21 – 49
- ⫽⫽ 6 – 20
- ▨ 50 +

Legende:

1. Peloponnes; E = Epidaurus
2. Attica
3. Thessaly
4. Asia; P = Pergamum
5. Aegean and Doric Islands; C = Cos
6. Thrace
7. Pontus
8. Italia
9. Gallia Narbonensis
10. Gallia Cisalpina
11. Gallia
12. Hispania
13. Britannia
14. Belgica
15. Germania inferior
16. Germania superior
17. Alps and Noricum
18. Pannonia superior
19. Pannonia inferior
20. Dalmatia
21. Dacia
22. Moesia superior
23. Macedonia
24. Epirus

25. Moesia inferior
26. Northern Black Sea
27. Sicilia
28. Sardinia
29. Africa
30. Mauretania
31. Numidia
32. Aegyptus
33. Cyrenaica
34. Galatia
35. Lycia and Pamphylia
36. Cappadocia
37. Cilicia
38. Media
39. Syria
40. Phoenicia
41. Judaea
42. Arabia

W = Brecon
N = Carpow
S = Memphis
E = Ecbatana

term 'plague' in this context – as Meier most recently did (1999) – is problematic because today the plague is seen as an infectious disease caused by the *Yersinia pestis* bacteria and applying the term in this context may be misunderstood as meaning that the epidemic of 430 BCE was indeed the same kind of disease. LEVEN quite rightly warns against such a retrospective diagnosis (2004 and 1997a: 13–15) in his history of infectious diseases. More recent genetic investigations into the measles virus, which was for a long time suspected to have caused the Athenian epidemic, prove that that virus is too recent (MANLEY 2014). So far it has only been possible to exclude some possible viruses, but none has as yet been confirmed. It was therefore certainly also the fear and the memory of that epidemic in Athens and its consequences, as well as the firm belief in its divine origin, that made the Athenians opt for Asclepius as a preventative measure (AUFFARTH 1995: 342–347, GARLAND 1992: 116–135, and SMARCZYK 1984: 245 ff.).

In 416/415 BCE, even before the Sicilian expedition, the Asclepieion was inaugurated on the southern slope of the Acropolis in Athens, above the theatre of Dionysus. There is evidence that the healing cult also flourished in the Greek communities of Egypt during that time, where it was either independent, as in the cities of Alexandria, Philadelphia, Oxyrhynchus, Hu and Menshiyeh, or conjoint with the sanctuaries of Imhotep, the Egyptian god of healing, as in Saqqara, Deir-el-Bahari, Deir-el-Medineh, and Phila. Although the two deities, Asclepius and Imhotep, have much in common, in terms of their origin and function, we must be careful not to conclude that they are identical (RÜTTIMANN 1986: 65–69, WILDUNG 1975, P. OXY. 1138 and 1381 with TOTTI-GEMÜND 1998). However, for Deir-el-Bahari ŁAJTAR (2006) presented the epigraphic evidence of inscriptions and ostraca, and he concluded that Imhotep was identified with Asclepius by the Greek community.

The sanctuary at Pergamum is the most prominent example for the first half of the fourth century BCE. PAUSANIAS has details of its foundation (2.26.8 with RADT 1999: 25 and 220–242). Archias, the son of Aristaichmus, is said to have introduced the Asclepian cult in Pergamum (MÜLLER 2011: 254–259). He was the first prytane of Pergamum and consequently a well-to-do and influential man. When hunting on mount Pindarus, Archias contracted an injury which was healed during his stay at Epidaurus. Full of gratitude he then brought the cult of Asclepius to Pergamum. The coins found at Pergamum are testimonies to the great importance of Asclepius (KRANZ 2004 and FRANKE 1969: 63). While in the fifth and fourth centuries BCE Apollo, as the city's first and foremost deity, appeared on the coins, it was Asclepius from the fourth century onward until the imperial period (AGELIDIS 2011: 174–183). The union of imperial cult and Asclepian piety secured the cult of Asclepius a secure position until the end of Antiquity. It was not until the sixth century CE that a Christian church was built in its place.

In the mid-fourth century BCE more settlements appeared in the eastern Aegean. An Asclepieion existed on the coast to the southwest of Delos, outside the city (KRUG 1993: 156 f.). The representatives of the *sui generis* scientific medicine, the Asclepiads, followed the tradition of the physicians from Cos. There was an Asclepieion on Cos, too, but not many remains are left that could provide information on its early period (INTERDONATO 2013 and KRUG 1993: 159–163). The first indications of its existence date from 411 BCE, when the island of Cos was devastated by an earthquake. The city was rebuilt with the addition of an Asclepieion which was completed in 366 BCE. The sanctuary, which was located in a cypress grove around two miles southwest of the city (KRUG 1993: 159–163), remained in use until it was destroyed in an earthquake in 511 CE. Between 1902 and 1904 the Asclepieion was excavated by the German archaeologist Rudolf Herzog (1871–1953). Italian archaeologists continued the excavations from 1912 to 1947 while the region was under Italian occupation. In 1928 restoration work was carried out. This Asclepieion has informed the modern image of the healing procedures applied on Cos. The most recent publication on the archaeology of the Coan Asclepieion is by INTERDONATO (2013).

This island is eminently important in the history of ancient medicine. Although an entire generation of physicians hailed from there, no clarity has as yet been gained, as SCHNALKE (1990: 19) points out, as to the relationship between the Hippocratic physicians and the cult and medicine of Asclepius. WICKKISER (2008) found a connection between the physicians and the Asclepieia in the fifth century BCE, but was unable to flesh his findings out convincingly. SCHNALKE's answer is only partly tenable because – although it is difficult to evaluate sources regarding the beginnings of medicine – the relationship in question can be defined more reliably for the imperial period. Based on a relief dedicated by a physician KRUG (1993: 152) derives that a good relationship existed between the Athenian sanctuary and the physicians and he assumes that this was also the case on Cos (KRUG 1993: 163). KRUG clearly follows HERZOG (1899/1931) here, who was convinced that the medical tradition in Cos reflected the true Asclepian temple medicine, but was unable to present evidence for his assumption.

Further settlements worth mentioning were in Bithynia, among them and above all the sanctuary at Prusa ad Olympum which also boasts ancient sulphurous thermal baths (KRUG 1993: 185, and further Asclepieia in EDELSTEIN/ EDELSTEIN 1945: 406–429). In the end Asclepius even spread to the Phoenicians, who equated him with the Phoenician deity Eshmun, to whom a temple from the fourth century BCE was consecrated in Sidon (see also STRAB. 17.3.4 on the consecration of the Eshmun Temple in Carthage in honour of Asclepius.) An epigraph is proof that Asclepius was worshipped in the temple of Sidon at that time (MC CASLAND 1939: 222). And there are other testimonies which prove Asclepius' penetration of the Phoenician culture. STRABO (16.2.22), for instance, referred to an Asclepian grove on the Tamyrus River, between Berytus and Sidon. PAUSANIAS (7.3.14) lets a Sidonian explain that they understood Asclepius and Apollo better than the Greeks.

Almost 200 cultic sites are documented for Asclepius by the end of the fourth century BCE (SCHNALKE 1990: 16 ff.). HART (2000: 165–182) devotes an entire chapter of his Asclepius monograph to the question as to how many Asclepieia existed in total. After evaluating the relevant secondary literature, he presents a table of his findings with 513 sites altogether. WALTON (1965) spoke of 368 settlements, having found numismatic references to 165. The diverging figures are mostly due to the criteria used to define an Asclepian site. HART's higher figure (2000) results mainly from the fact that he includes remote numismatic material too. SCHÄFER (2000: 261) speaks of 411 Asclepian sites for the whole of antiquity, but fails to mention how he has arrived at this figure. Most recently RIETHMÜLLER (2005: 75 f.) counted 159 cultic sites for mainland Greece. He speaks of 192 definite Asclepieia outside mainland Greece and another 44 for which there was no conclusive evidence. Outside the Greek territory RIETHMÜLLER (2005: 85), who bases his conclusions on the list provided by WALTON (1965), assumes 409 definite and 77 possible cultic sites.

At the beginning of the third century BCE the Asclepian cult arrived in Rome (LIV. 10.47.7 and OV. met. 15.622–744). As in the case of Apollo Medicus, the transfer of his mythical son Asclepius and the Asclepian healing cult to Rome was prompted by an epidemic (HAEHLING VON LANZENAUER 1996: 18–24, KRUG 1993: 163–165, GRAF 1992b: 160–167, DE FILIPPIS CAPPAI 1991, ROESCH 1982, BECHER 1970: 217–228, SCARBOROUGH 1969: 66–75, and KERÉNYI 1956: 4–16). Rome was engaged in warfare with the Samnites when, in 293 BCE, a group of senators was instructed by the Sibyls to travel to Epidaurus because a highly contagious epidemic was raging in Latium (BIRABEN 1996: 377 f.). Epidemics were seen as punishments sent by the gods for human failings. Oracles, miracle-workers (male and female!) were consulted on ways of pacifying the displeased deity (HORSTMANSHOFF 1992). When the delegates returned they brought with them a serpent which they released near the river Tiber. The snake slipped into the water and determined where Asclepius was to be worshipped by settling on Tiber Island. In this cultural transfer the serpent symbolizes Asclepius and his healing cult, as is apparent from the transfer by chariot to Athens and Sicyon, and by boat to Epidaurus Limera and Rome, and finally to Pergamum (SCHNALKE 2005, CLINTON 1994, and HAFNER 1990). A Roman medallion from the mid-second century CE commemorates the event (fig. 2). The bronze medallion depicts the reception of the serpent of Asclepius in Rome and on Tiber Island, as well as a bridge and a boat. Asclepius receives the serpent in person as it arrives after its voyage from Epidaurus to Tiber Island.

In memory of the serpent's voyage the island was remodelled to resemble a stone ship (fig. 7 and PFEFFER 1969: 22–27 and 98–102). The downstream end of Tiber Island still boasts remnants of the shiplike stone structures (KRAUSS 1944). Tiber Island is joined to the mainland by two bridges, *Pons Fabricius* and *Pons Cestius*. The island has solid foundations which constitute the ship's floor. At the ship's prow stands the temple of Asclepius, at its stern a temple of Jupiter. To the left of the bow we still see a relief showing the bust of Asclepius and the serpent wound around the rod next to him (fig. 9 a/b). Tiber Island has retained its medical tradition to this day: in 1582 the Hospitaller Order of St. John of God founded a hospital there that still exists today.

A cultic site for Asclepius was erected on Tiber Island and the sanctuary was inaugurated in 291 BCE. The cultic forms remained the same as those of the major sanctuaries in Greece and Asia Minor (FEST. p. 268 L.). As early as the second century BCE, Asclepius and Apollo had attained the same rank as the Roman goddess Salus (LIV. 4.37.2), which is proof that, in their search for new religious affiliations, the Romans were convinced by the healer and saviour Asclepius and decided to include this eminent representative of the Greek healing deities into the Roman state cult (LIV. 10.47.7, VAL. MAX. 1.8.2, OROS. 3.22.5 f., and BECHER 1970: 219 f.). This step marked the actual beginning of Rome's medical history.

Tiber Island soon became a refuge for the weak and sick. Slaves who had become infirm and could no longer work were shunted off to the island by their masters (KRUG 1993: 164). The poorest of the poor were offered 'asylum' in the Asclepieion. Claudius had enacted a law that guaranteed slaves their freedom if they were released in the sacred precinct of Tiber Island (SUET. Claud. 25.2, DIOD. 60.29.7 and DIG. 40.8.2). It usually fell to the emperors to look after the needs and concerns of these healing centres (ZIETHEN 1994: 178 with note 38 f.). The fact that the slaves were left on the island suggests that they received medical treatment free of charge. It is not possible to reconstruct what other kinds of supplicant came to Tiber Island. The emperors hardly ever took notice of the local Asclepieion. Like other well-to-do Romans they went to Greece or Asia Minor for medical consultations, to Pergamum, for instance, or to Abonotteichos (Ionopolis) in Paphlagonia (STEGER 2005a, NUTTON 2004, 282 f., and BECHER 1970: 243).

During the imperial period the cult of Asclepius spread further and further from its original centre (HAEHLING VON LANZENAUER 1996: 24–27). From the first century CE the cult is also documented in Palestine, where it is linked to the hot springs near Tiberias. Coins from Tiberias, dating back to between 99 and 108 CE, show the bust of Trajan on one side and Hygieia with the serpent, sitting above a spring, on the other (MC CASLAND 1939: 224). It is not possible to derive conclusions on any healing activities from these testimonies. In the late first or early second century CE, Antoninus Pius ordered the minting of coins that depicted Asclepius and Hygieia together (KRANZ 2010: 71–91 and MC CASLAND 1939: 225). Starting with the Severan dynasty, Aesculapius and Salus (or Hygieia) were regularly depicted on the imperial mintage (FRANKE 1969: 66). If she is not depicted with the typical attributes or in the presence of Asclepius, Hygieia is difficult to identify on coins or sculptures (KRANZ 2010: 71 f.). Right up into the imperial period Hygieia had no cult of her own (RIETHMÜLLER 2005: II 253) but shared a temple with Asclepius, as in Pergamum for instance (KRANZ 2010: 93).

The cult flourished from the second century CE onward. RÜTTIMANN (1986) explored its golden age in his dissertation, paying particular attention to its influence on early Christianity. The cult's importance is reflected in the vast additions made to it, starting with the reign of Emperor Trajan, and in the lasting presence (which is certainly documented for Asia Minor) of Asclepius – or Aesculapius – on the gold, silver, or bronze coins of the Roman emperors (KRANZ 1990: 130 and FRANKE 1969: 66 f.). In a speech he made in front of the Emperor Antoninus Pius in Rome, the orator Aelius Aristides said that all the cities of Greece were flourishing under Roman rule (ARISTEID. or. 26.94–96). Coastline and country were richly strewn with cities promoted by the Romans. Aristides compared Rome's keen commitment to the Greeks with the care foster parents devote to their children by holding a protective hand over them. While Aristides' speech is embellished and exaggerated as becomes a proper eulogy, it nonetheless conveys the message that the provinces were thriving under Roman stewardship. While the Greeks always measured their status quo against their glorious past and while they were aware of certain material and political deficits (URSIN 2014: 56–60), the cities of Asia

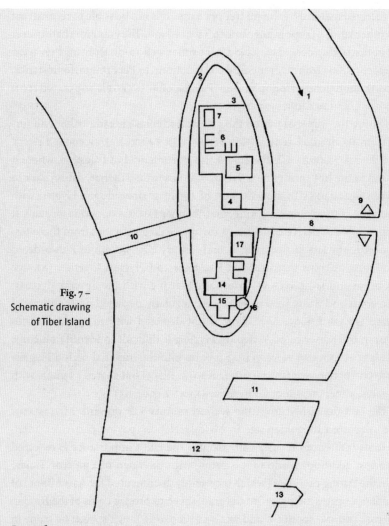

Fig. 7 –
Schematic drawing
of Tiber Island

Legend:

1. Tiber with direction of flow
2. Insula
3. Present-day hospital
4. Modern pharmacy
5. Courtyard with fountain
6. Modern stairway surrounded by temple walls
7. Corridor leading to diagnostic imaging department with temple walls visible below
8. Pons Fabricius
9. Statue of Janus
10. Pons Cestius
11. Pons Aemilius
12. Modern bridge
13. Cloaca maxima
14. Church of San Bartolomeo
15. Site of the healing spring of the temple of Aesculapius
16. Remains of the prow of the ship-shaped temple of Aesculapius
17. Site of ancient Jewish hospital

Minor in particular benefited from the euergetism of the emperor and the local elites, and they thrived economically as well as culturally. The Emperor Hadrian himself visited Asia Minor several times on his extensive travels. In 124 CE he came to the *provincia Asia* for the first time, and again on his second great journey, on which he embarked in 128 CE. Hadrian clearly made every effort on these excursions to show how much he cared for his entire empire (LE GLAY 1978). Achaea and Asia Minor benefited from his benevolence which manifested in the founding of cities, in building activities, and other forms of support (PAUS. 1.5.5; 1.20.7 and 1.36.3). And the local populations, displaying a propagandist and ideological reflex, showed their gratitude by devoting inscriptions and coins to him (CHRIST 1995: 319–321). Hadrian made noticeable efforts with his religious policies to guide the various populations toward one dominating deity (KRANZ 1990: 125 f.). He knew like no other Roman emperor how to use religion as a means of asserting his own political interests.

The sanctuary at Pergamum was widely changed and promoted after the late first century CE (ZIEGENAUS 1981), as is documented in dedications from that time (KRUG 1993: 166, KRANZ 1990: 134 f., and HABICHT 1969). The senators L. Cuspius Pactumeius Rufinus (HALFMANN 1979, Nr. 66) and A. Claudius Charax (HALFMANN 1979, No. 73 and HABICHT 1959/60) both made important donations to the Asclepieion. Rufinus dedicated the round temple of Zeus to Asclepius Soter (ARISTEID. hier. log. 4.28. GAL. De anat. admin. 2.224 f. K. and PETSALIS-DIOMIDIS 2010: 194–202) and Charax contributed to the propylon at the Asclepieion (HABICHT 1969, No. 141).

Pergamum produced its own series of coins, depicting Asclepius with Telesphorus and an omphalos (KAMPMANN 1992/3: 42, and generally on the Pergamene Asclepius coins, KRANZ 2004: 98–131). AELIUS ARISTIDES (hier. log. 2.10; 3.23 and 4.16) mentioned a statue of Telesphorus in the temple of Hygieia who, in the imperial period, was always worshipped together with Asclepius (KRANZ 2010: 110–162). The significance of the omphalos, a sphere located at the lower end of Asclepius' robe, is discussed controversially (HERRMANN 1959). The theory that the omphalos symbolizes Asclepius' heroic status is compelling since it is clearly associated with the mortuary cult and with hero worship. The Pergamene coins depict the Amelung-type Asclepius which is also known from a statue donated to Pergamum by Hadrian (KRANZ 1990: 130 f.). While Asclepius has appeared in various forms on emissions from Asia Minor since late Hellenistic times, the new Amelung type became prevalent from the Hadrianic era onward (KAMPMANN 1992/3 and KRANZ 2004: 38). It can be said to have played a particular part in Hadrian's religious policy (AMANDRY 1993). Even the mintage in Hadrian's early years as emperor discloses his political program in concepts such as piety, harmony, justice, outer and inner peace, unity and, finally, the striving for a golden age (BMC III 278, No. 312, pl. 52.10 and RIC 136), while Antoninus Pius simply continued this approach. A veritable city culture unfolded with the building of new temple complexes, halls, streets, gymnasiums, thermal baths and ports (JONES 1971 and DRÄGER 1993).

Apart from the groups of physicians that are obvious representatives of the medical market (II.3), and the non-medical groups which, at second glance, also appear to belong to it (II.5), there were also magic and religion as influential elements in the sphere of healing: the Roman Empire was tolerant and patient when it came to polytheistic approaches. Beliefs focused on the theocracy. This created a backdrop which offered space for omens, magic and miracles (CHRIST 1995: 564 ff.). Supported by the growing influence of the magic world, Alexander of Abonuteichos was able to assume the role of a prophet and declare himself to be the representative of the god Glycon. This god was the 'new Asclepius', and oracles and mysteries were devoted to him. In the second half of the second century CE this cult became widespread in Asia Minor, Thrace, and Rome and was able to survive into the third century CE (LUCIAN. Alex. 10 and STEGER 2005a: 8 f.). The Roman satirists could hardly restrain their scorn at such a development (IUV. 6.549 ff.). It is therefore not surprising that the magical concept of healing added another aspect to the medical marketplace.

Although LUCIAN's 'Alexander' (around 180 CE) provides some information on the relationship between the healing cult and the worship of Asclepius, the Asclepian medicine practised in Abonuteichus in Asia Minor remains rather unclear (STEGER 2005a). LANGHOLF (1996) has demonstrated that, while Lucian's medical knowledge met the imperial requirements and while he was interested in medicine over and above those standards, he was not as advanced as the contemporary specialist literature. Lucian's relationship with medicine seems complex because of the literary form he used. Although he concentrates on unmasking Alexander's questionable oracular activity (VICTOR 1997: 3 and 15), some aspects of medical practice can be gleaned from his work (LUCIAN. Alex. 22).

Τοὺς δὲ ἀπέτρεπεν ἢ προὔτρεπεν, ὡς ἂν ἄμεινον ἔδοξεν αὐτῷ εἰκάζοντι· τοῖς δὲ θεραπείας προὔλεγεν καὶ διαίτας, εἰδώς, ὅπερ ἐν ἀρχῇ ἔφην, πολλὰ καὶ χρήσιμα φάρμακα. μάλιστα δὲ εἰδοκίμουν παρ' αὐτῷ αἱ κυτμίδες, ἀκόπου τι ὄνομα πεπλασμένον, ἐκ λίπους ἀρκείου συντεθειμένου.

He advised some in favour and others against a particular action, as he saw fit. For others again he prescribed medical treatment because, as I said from the start, he knew many useful remedies. He was particularly fond of 'cytmides', a phantasy name for a tonic made of bear's fat.

More detailed information on forms of treatment and on diets is missing, and one is left asking where Alexander had come by his medical knowledge. According to Lucian he was the student of an unnamed man from Tyana who was close to the well-known miracle-worker Apollonius (LUCIAN. Alex. 5), a fact that associated him with the contemporary quackery which he criticized vehemently in his dialog *Philopseudes*. No conclusions can be derived as to his affiliation to a particular medical tradition. Lucian does provide some details concerning the cult in Abonuteichus, however, saying, for instance, that Alexander deposited a goose egg, which he had emptied before and into which he had placed a newborn snake, into the foundations of the temple (LUCIAN. Alex. 13). Instead of the cult being transferred, as happened in 420 and 293 BCE to Athens and Rome respectively, the snake in this case was 'born' in the sanctuary. Egg and serpent are both well-known attributes of Asclepius (fig. 5 and SCHNALKE 2005).

Research tends to assign the magic healing practices to the sphere of religious-magic medicine (HOHEISEL 1995). Generally, it needs to be considered that religion and magic intermingled in everyday life and that they are therefore difficult to separate from one another (ZIETHEN 1994: 175 and PETZOLDT 1978). This was true for the Greek culture in particular because all the Greek gods possessed healing powers. Amynus, the hero Iatrus, Aristomachus and his father, Amphiaraos, are good examples. Religious approaches to healing therefore have a long history (NUTTON 1999b: 1110 f.). Even ancient Babylon had *magi* who emphasized the filiation of their doctrine, as did the early Greek physicians (BURKERT 1984: 43 ff.).

Magic was the art of the μάγοι, who had been known as such since the late sixth century BCE (GRAF 1996: 24–57). The term derives from the Persian word for 'priest' or for a person concerned with religious matters (GRAF 1996: 24). Other terms include καθάρται for purifiers, and ἀγύρται for mendicants (HIPP. Morb. Sacr. 2 (6.352 f. L.)). 'Magia' and 'magus', moreover, are loan words from the Greek which first appear in Latin in the writings of Catullus and Cicero. (CIC. leg. 2.26 and CATULL. 90). Information on magic activities can also be found on imperial papyri from Egypt, which mention pathogenic spells (*defixiones*) and amulets against diseases. It is said, for instance, that a magic doll caused a plague (GRAF 1992a). Sexual disorders in particular were explained in this way (OV. AM. 3.7.27–29 and GRAF 1996: 128). The papyri also include collections of magical recipes and ritual instructions for magicians, which range all the way from home remedies for headaches and coughs to drugs that bring about hallucinatory dreams, to prescriptions that can appease the wrath of an employer or win the heart of a woman. The Greek magical papyri have been collected by PREISENDANZ (PGM) and published by HEIN-RICHS (1974) in a second, new edition. A complete overview was presented by BRASHEAR (1995). On magic practices in ancient Egypt in general up to early Christianity KÁKOSY's monograph (1989) is best consulted. Magical effects were also attributed to the curse tablets (*defixionum tabellae*), tin sheets with inscriptions aimed to destroy the health of the cursed person for good (STAM-ATU 2005). All the ancient spell tablets that have been preserved are included in the database of the TheDeMa project (*Thesaurus Defixionum Magdeburgensis*) at the Otto-von-Guericke-University in Magdeburg, Germany.

> natam primum e medicina nemo dubitabit ac specie salutari increpsisse velut al-tiorem sanctioremque medicinam, ita blandissimis desideratissimisque promissis addidisse vires religionis, ad quas maxime etiam nunc caligat humanum genus (…). No one will doubt that it [magic] first originated in medicine and that, under the plausible guise of promoting health, it insinuated itself among humankind as a higher and more sacred branch of the medical art, by attributing to the most seduc-tive and desired promises religious powers which to the present day keep human-kind in the dark (…). (PLIN. nat. 30.2)

Pliny sees magic as a combination of medicine, religion, and astrology (PLIN. nat. 30.1). He differentiates between good and efficient medical practice, which he calls *medicina*, and the false and presumptuous *magia*, which is lofty and of divine origin. Pliny is not altogether consistent, however, since he recommends *magorum remedia* elsewhere for cases where all other attempts have failed (STANNARD 1987). This view places Pliny on a par with those who consider magical intervention to be appropriate in two instances: firstly, when sickness and death occur unexpectedly and inexplicably, and secondly, in cases of professional failure (GRAF 1996: 151). Amulets were seen as helpful in cases of epilepsy, fever, toothache, headache or painful limbs, a condition Libanius endured repeatedly (KOTANSKY 1991). In both cases there are no ra-tional explanations and magic is therefore indicated.

The activities of magicians and miracle workers were strictly divided from the other approaches to healing (HIPPOKR. Morb. Sacr. 1. SOPH. Ai. 581 f. ULP. Digest. 50.13.3, and KUDLIEN 1988/1983). The fact remains, however, that it is sometimes difficult to draw the line between the two (LLOYD 1979). Many physicians were knowledgeable astrologists (PTOL. Tetr. 16 f., HEPH. Astr. praef. (Egypt), and CAT. COD. ASTROL. GRAEC. 5.4.172.7–12 (Cod. Vatic.)), while the *magi*, on the other hand, also had medical duties (PLIN. nat. 29.53; 29.68 and LUCIAN. Alex. 5 f.).

A high degree of magic and mystery was assigned to the Jewish population: aside from the Jewish physicians there were also Jewish faith healers at work, constituting a link to the Jewish miracle-rabbis. KUDLIEN (1985) concentrates in his study on the primarily non-Jewish territories of the Roman Empire and omits Judea and Palestine. ALLAN (2001) looks at the status and role of physicians in ancient Israel up until 70 CE, and particularly their demarcation from religion and magic. In late antiquity the interwovenness of medicine and religion became apparent in the fact that Jewish – like Christian – priests could also be physicians (JACOBOVITS 1959: 239–241). It is therefore not surprising that not much of a difference was made between the two groups (APUL. apol. 43 and LUCIAN. Alex. passim). Yet, the phenomenon is the more unexpected seeing that in theory there had been a clear differentiation since the first century CE (PLIN. nat. 30.1 ff. and APUL. apol. 43). It can be concluded that the *magi* occupied a particular position in the health market, just as magicians did in primitive cultures, and that their activities were ritualistic. Unlike the ordinary cults, which relied on groups, the *magus* performed his rituals in isolation. Whether this also applies to the cultic aspects of medicine needs to be critically investigated (GRAF 1996: 204).

Propitiatory inscriptions found in Asia Minor from the first to the third centuries CE document magical and religious approaches to medicine. PETZL (1994) produced an annotated collection of sources on this topic. Propitiatory inscriptions are expressions of cultic purity. They provide an insight into medical elements rather than a specific and uniform medical concept (CHANIOTIS 1995). Aside from the usual prayer and sacrifice they constitute a further, separate form of cult (GRAF 1998: 246). Most of these sources reflect a particular local character and religious approach. CHANIOTIS (1995) points out that these inscriptions epitomize the presence of medical knowledge in the remote regions of Asia Minor, with some cases expressing a clear dualism of medical and divine elements. Devotees typically feel ill because they have sinned against a deity. This causal relationship between 'sin' and illness is also important for the medical market. While illness arises as a consequence of sin, the confessing of sins is a prerequisite for recovery (VON SIEBENTHAL 1950). KUDLIEN (1978) finds no signs of forced confessions in the Iamata of Asclepius collected by EDELSTEIN/EDELSTEIN (1945). KUDLIEN (1978: 4–6) is therefore reluctant to assign to the Asclepian cult the characteristic sequence of sin, sickness, punishment, and confession. The Iamata speak neither of sins nor the confession of sins. With the emergence of Christianity, theologians began to instrumentalize this link by correlating sickness with sin. Medicines were replaced by prayer and confession (JAMES 5.14–16). The miraculous healings described in hagiographic texts, however, go further than prayer and confession. Gregory of Tours, for instance, relates how the eyesight of the deacon Theumoder was miraculously restored (GREG. TUR. Mart. 2.19).

Propitiatory inscriptions found in Phrygia and Lydia often mention gynaecological or ophthalmological problems. One documented example of eye problems stems from the sanctuary of the local deities Anaitis and Men Tiamu, in the region of Kula. (PETZL 1994: 10–21 No. 70). It is a pedimental stele made of white marble with acroteria and a tenon, adorned with an image that shows, from left to right, two busts, a right leg with a foot on a ledge and a pair of eyes. The inscription below reads "The wrath of the Goddess Anaitis and of Men Tiamu was appeased by these sacrifices." While cause and aim of this wrath are not explained, the image shows the body parts that were its targets. Blindness is a punishment typically inflicted by the gods, but pathophysiological causes also need to be considered, that is, a chronic condition for which neither a quick recovery nor a quick death was to be expected. Only divine intervention could help in such a case. A refusal to help from the god in question could be interpreted as a further punishment of the sinner. While this example contains no medical reference, it nonetheless documents a local medical cult in the imperial period. Under certain circumstances patients seemed to have felt safer in the hands of a god than in those of another representative of the medical profession.

The cult of Asclepius was a potential threat for Christianity and its claim to exclusivity (HAEHLING VON LANZENAUER 1996: 3 ff. and RENGSTORFF 1953). RÜTTIMANN (1986: 128–178 and 179–211) referred to devotional objects to illustrate the influence of the Asclepian cult on early Christianity in the second century CE. Due to the tolerance of the Adoptive Emperors, Christianity was able to grow and become established during their period. But once the imperial cult had allied itself with the Asclepian piety Asclepius became a real danger for Christianity. Jesus Christ, the performer of miracles and miracle healings, became a rival of Asclepius (VON STADEN 1998). It is interesting that there are many parallels between the myth surrounding Asclepius and the life of Christ, in particular the fact that they both died violent deaths as human beings and that this circumstance contributed to the trust invested in them (STEGER 2000: 37 and BECHER 1970: 249–255). Eusebius doubts the divine nature of Asclepius and sees him as purely human (EUS. Pr. Ev. 3.14.13 and LEVEN 1987: 142 ff.). This similarity between Asclepius and Christ in pictorial representations remains a striking feature (KRUG 1993: 128) until late antiquity.

The extensive branching out of the Asclepius cult was the greatest obstacle for Christianity. There were a great number of Asclepian sanctuaries in Laconia, for instance (WIDE 1973: 182–186). Four sanctuaries are documented in Sparta alone: Asclepius Cotyleus on the road to Therapne (PAUS. 3.19.7), the shrine "near the Agiads" (PAUS. 3.14.2), the sanctuary of Asclepius Agnitas (PAUS. 3.14.7) and the famous site next to the Booneta (PAUS. 3.15.10). There is documentation of a certain Pomponia Callistonice, a priestess of the sanctuary of Asclepius Schoinatas in Elos on the southern coast of Laconia (IG 602.10 f. and HUPFLOHER 2000: 81–84). During the "imperial crisis" of the third century CE (WITSCHEL 1999 and STROBEL 1993) the Asclepian sanctuaries were particularly popular.

In the fall of 214 CE, the Emperor Caracalla came to Pergamum in order to recover from an illness he had contracted in Nicomedia (HEROD. 4.7.1; 4.8.3; 4.10.1–11. SHA Carac. 6.1–6, CASS. DIO 78.15.2–6 and ROBERT 1973/1978). For this visit he had ordered the temple of Asclepius in Pergamum to be renovated (PRICE 1984: 152 f.), and he gave permission for the image of Asclepius with the omphalos (and Telesphorus), an well-known Pergamene image, to be used as a motif on Roman imperial coins. Up until the second century CE Asclepius had hardly been depicted on any imperial emissions (KRANZ 1990: 129 f. incl. footnote 21, and 145 with footnote 125). The first time Asclepius appeared on a coin was on a small gold piece, where one can just make out the round shape known as omphalos close to his cloak. One year later, Asclepius appeared with the omphalos and with Telesphorus on coins of all nominal values (MATTINGLY/CARSON/HILL 1975 No. 148, 278–280, 291, 292–297). In this context, Asclepius of Pergamum was venerated as *deus Pergameus* (MART. 11.16.2 and KRANZ 2004). One year later, in 215 CE, Caracalla sacrificed to Asclepius in Aegeae – as Alexander the Great had once done in Soli (ARR. an. 2.5.5 and CURT. 3.7.2). Having successfully fought the Cilicians in the surrounding mountains, Alexander had returned to Soli where he honoured a pledge he had made when he fell ill, namely to sacrifice to Asclepius. He held a great parade with a torchlight procession and athletic and musical competitions (ROBERT 1973: 199 f.). Alexander had contact with Asclepius several times, for instance during his campaign at Ecbatana (ARR. an. 7.14.5 f.). And lastly, there is evidence of Alexander making votive offerings at the sanctuary in Gortys (PAUS. 8.28.1). Caracalla was so keen to copy Alexander and his political program that it came close to an obsession (BIRLEY 1997: 189 f.). How seriously he took this, is apparent from his behaviour in Alexandria in 215 CE, where the population mocked him for his veneration of Alexander. Caracalla revenged himself by gathering the young Alexandrian recruits, whom he had intended to take with him, and by having them killed by his own people (CHRIST 1995: 622 f.).

Aegeae was an important city because of its geographical situation as a hub between Syria and Cilicia. The Asclepian shrine at Aegeae was famous far beyond the city and was in no way inferior to the great healing sites at Cos, Pergamum and Epidaurus (WEISS 1982: 198 ff.). The city had traditional links with the Greek and the Roman Alexander. The Emperor Severus Alexander was honoured at Aegeae, as is apparent from the fact that the city adopted the epithet Alexandropoulis and also from the devotional objects that have been preserved. An inscription on an altar in Aegeae dating back to 238 CE empha-sizes the city's dedication to the deified Severan dynasty, mentioning Alexan-der in particular (WEISS 1982). This dedication also extends to the city's two demigods, Asclepius and Hygieia, who are also honoured on other imperial monuments found in Aegeae (ROBERT 1973: 101). Aegeae had boasted a tem-ple to Asclepius since late Hellenistic times (ZIEGLER 1994: 200). Alexander Severus had visited the city and its Asclepieion and awarded it a neokorate, an act which signified that Aegeae was now, with Tarsos and Anazarbus, the site of a provincial imperial temple with all the corresponding institutions, including the *Agones* (HERZ 1997). The neokorate was reflected in the city's title and mintage, which were both means of self-representation. The coins of Aegeae prove that several emperors maintained a very close connection with the city, in particular with the sanctuary of Asclepius. There are coins of the Emperor Valerian which depict an imperial bust in conjunction with the rod of Asclepius. The Emperor is shown to be a great devotee to the Asclepius of Aegeae because he is even depicted with Asclepius' attributes. Similar coins exist of Severus Alexander, also depicting an imperial bust with the attributes of Asclepius. The coins for Severus Alexander only refer to the neokorate after 231/232 CE, a fact which seems to indicate that the granting of the neokorate to Aegeae was associated with the sojourn of Severus Alexander in this city. The same applies to the coins that link Severus Alexander with Asclepius. It seems that the Asclepian sanctuary was at the same time Aegeae's neokorate temple. The sanctuary of Asclepius was so rich in tradition and so important that its advancement to a neokorate temple was not called into question. Un-der Decius, whose religious policy included the promotion of traditional cults (ZIEGLER 1994: 199, 201–204), the positive relationship between the emperor and Asclepius was apparent from the fact that Aegeae was given the epithet 'Asclepioupolis' rather than the more likely 'Decianoi'.

Asclepius and his healing cult were consequently highly esteemed in the midst of the 'imperial crisis' of the third century CE. Christian tradition, on the other hand, as described by Eusebius, Origen and Celsus, no longer considered Asclepius to be *primus inter pares* but identified him as the leading representative of the pagan cults. The fact of Asclepius' obvious promotion through Decius' religious policy proves this emperor's hostility toward Christianity (ZIEGLER 1994: 204 f.). His favouring of the Asclepian temple at Aegeae as a supranational sanctuary is in itself an unmistakable sign of this antagonism. The city of Aegeae, as is apparent from its superior infrastructure, also benefited from this imperial preference. The healing cult itself contributed the economic means for this development, because the cities with major Asclepian sanctuaries derived considerable income from their operation (ZIEGLER 1994: 206). DREXHAGE (1981: 19–26) examines the relationship between the pagan-religious life and economic structures. The fact that cultic sites generally had an impact on a city's economic situation led CASTRITIUS (1973) to point out that the commercial aspects of ancient religiousness were threatened by the persistent diffusion of Christianity. Christians were therefore disliked not least because their growing strength spelt the decline of the cities' healing cults and consequently endangered the foundations of their existence (ZIEGLER 1994: 207 with note 102).

As a result of these serious circumstances, Asclepius was exposed to increasing and ever more vigorous attacks (TEMKIN 1991: 94 ff.). Christ was presented as the true redeemer and healer (IUST. Mart. apol. 1.21 and TERT. nat. 2.14.13) while Asclepius was denounced as a mercenary physician (ἰατρὸς φιλάργυρος). CLEMENS of Alexandria (Protr. 2.30.1 f.) pointed out that Christian physicians did not accept money (ἀνάργυροι) in return for their services (KOETTING 1980: 204). The physicians/faith healers Cosmas and Damian are said to have died as martyrs, at Aegeae of all places, during the persecution of Christians under Diocletian (ZIEGLER 1994: 210 with note 117) and to have become revered saints there in the third and fourth centuries CE. This veneration continued with Saint Thalelaius who had become a renowned healer at Aegeae (ZIEGLER 1994: 211 incl. note 12). These circumstances explain Eusebius' comment that the Emperor Constantine ordered the destruction of the sanctuary at Aegeae in 331 CE. Eusebius thought that the emperor acted justly when he decreed that the temple should be levelled to the ground, because he obeyed the rightful God and true redeemer (EUS. Vita Const. 3.56.1 f., ZIEGLER 1994: 207 f., LEVEN 1987: 152 f. and ROBERT 1973: 188 ff.). The destruction of a pagan sanctuary is in direct opposition to Constantine's view on cults and holy sites, however. And it would, moreover, have been impossible to simply destroy a sanctuary of such monumental dimensions. Only a year earlier Constantine had himself portrayed as *sol invictus* in the newly founded Constantinople. It is hardly conceivable that Constantine would have himself depicted as a pagan deity in a city founded by him whilst giving orders to demolish the highly esteemed sanctuary of an influential pagan half-god. Throughout his reign, Constantine's religious policy was markedly tolerant and integrative: he held on to the pagan cults whilst also supporting and favouring Christianity (CLAUSS 1997b: 292–297). In his comments Eusebius tried to give the impression that Constantine followed the advice of his political and religious counsellor in this instance, which aimed at preventing the further polarization of Asclepius' cult and Christianity. What really lies behind Eusebius' comment is his biased intention to present Christ as victorious. His account is therefore to be seen as Christian propaganda and the attempt to present Christianity as superior to, and truer than, the pagan religion (EUS. Pr. Ev. 5.1.15). Eusebius' version of events is therefore unsuitable for reconstructing who commissioned the destruction of the sanctuary at Aegeae in 311 CE. ZIEGLER (1994: 208) explains the destruction in the light of the political and military conflict between Constantine and Licinius in the years leading up to 324 CE. Because Licinius ruled over the east, where Aegeae was situated (LIB. or. 306), the Asclepian sanctuary was destroyed for political, religious and socio-economic reasons after Constantine's victory. It was an act of revenge of the followers of Christ against the pagans and the city of Aegeae.

The destruction of the Asclepieion at Aegeae does not signify the end of the Asclepian cult any more than the end of Aegeae spelt the end of the Asclepian cult within the Empire in general. A votive inscription from Epidaurus, for instance, attests to a continued cult to Asclepius Aegeotes (355 CE) at Aegeae (IG IV² 438 and ROBERT 1973: 193). The religious life in the Empire continued to straddle the dualism of Christianity and paganism, a fact that again is proof that the emergence of Christianity was a drawn-out process and that it is too much of a simplification to say that the downfall of paganism was directly followed by the rise of Christianity.

The period was moreover determined by internal Christian as well as Christian-pagan conflicts. Constantius II, the son of Emperor Constantine and ruler over the entire empire from the summer of 353 CE, turned away from the old gods. He was committed to Arianism and pursued a militant anti-pagan policy which he relinquished when visiting Rome in 357 CE (AMM. 16.10.1–17), because he could not disregard Rome's pagan past during his visit.

His successor Julian, whose philosophical studies had awakened his interest in paganism/polytheism (WIEMER 1997: 334 f.), saw the elevation of Christianity and the forsaking of the pagan healing cults as the beginning of a process of decline. Julian the Apostate did therefore everything in his power to restore paganism, and as the sole Augustus, he made it his mission (from 361 CE) to set the whole world free from the fetters of the false creed and to set humanity back on the right path. In his forced attempts at repaganization Julian was guided by the Roman sun god *Sol Invictus* (IUL. epist. 111 Bidez). The fact that Apollo was also revered as a sun god, boded well for his mythical son Asclepius. Julian aligned his comprehensive reform activities with his religious and cultural policies. He had the temples of the ancient Gods restored or newly built, gave land back that had been confiscated by the Christians, and prohibited the building of new Christian churches. He created a confrontational climate that aggravated internal Christian tensions as well as the conflict between pagans and Christians. Julian did all he could to replace the Christian god with a pagan deity and, as part of these aspirations, the cult of Asclepius was to be extended from an individualized to a universal religion of salvation. Julian saw Asclepius as the deity that held out a rescuing right hand to the entire world (ZIETHEN 1994: 185). When Julian was killed in the summer of 363 CE during his Persian campaign, his forced policy of repaganization also came to an end: no ruler after him would return to it. Even his direct successor, Jovian, was a Christian who undid most of the religious-political changes introduced by Julian (AMM. 25.2.5 f.).

The Emperor Valentinian, who ruled after the death of Jovian (364 CE), tolerated the pagan cults (AMM. 30.9.5), but his brother Valens favoured the Christian religion. Valens governed in the east and shared the religious-political ideas of Constantinus II. And yet, the cult of Asclepius survived even these tumultuous times. The sanctuary at Tarsus, for instance, was very much frequented even after the death of Julian and up until the reign of Emperor Valens (LIB. op. 695; 706; 1286; 1300; 1303). Emperor Theodosius I. made the Nicene Christian creed the state religion in the Roman Empire. In 380 CE he issued an edict at Thessaloniki that was to strengthen the unity of Christians in the Nicene Creed. In the same year the edict was confirmed at the Council of Constantinople and Christianity was declared the state religion (COD. THEOD. 16.1.2). Theodosius refused the title *pontifex maximus*, rejected the traditional cults, and pursued a decidedly anti-pagan course politically. In 392 CE, he issued a decree from Milan to the prefect of Rome forbidding the practice of pagan cults in the entire Roman Empire. His son Arcadius would later order countless pagan sanctuaries to be destroyed (COD. THEOD. 16.10.16). In the first half of the fifth century CE Christianity prevailed, but the cult of Asclepius retained its importance. Emperor Justinian's appeal to all pagans in 529 CE to embrace Christianity was contemporary with the sanctuary of Asclepius at Ascalon (Phoenicia). Proclus, one if not the last of the classical philosophers in Athens, composed a hymn to Asclepius Leontouchos of Ascalon, which has not been preserved but has been transmitted indirectly in other accounts. It proves that the sanctuary of Asclepius existed into the sixth century CE. Asclepius and his cult therefore represent a Greco-Roman tradition that survived the transition from late antiquity to the early Middle Ages and preserved the memory of ancient times.

III.2 – The sites of Asclepian healing

Research defines the relationship between religion and medicine as a religious-magical medicine carried out by magicians in healing cults. In addition to this, it says, there is a rational-scientific medicine based on nature observation and a rational understanding of nature. Two ways of practising medicine are being differentiated here: the rational-scientific approach presented in the specialist literature, which is associated with the names of Hippocrates and Galen, and the (numinous) religious-magical approach that is seen as relying on the potency of religion in the ancient lifeworld (SCHUBERT/HUTTNER 1999: 436, KRUG 1993: 120 ff. and RÜTTIMANN 1986). There is no competition, we are told, between these two forms of medicine: it is more like a coexistence of religious and profane medicine (SCHUBERT/HUTTNER 1999: 486 f.). While STROHMAIER (1996: 164 f.) proposes that the two coexisted peacefully, SCHÄFER (2000: 264 ff.) compares them without taking into account that the kind of medicine described in the Hippocratic Corpus does not reflect the everyday practice and that its comparison with the everyday practice of Asclepian medicine, as it is portrayed in the relevant inscriptions, can only be flawed.

The prevailing view has so far been that the two forms of medicine existed peacefully alongside each other. This is surprising and it needs to be critically investigated whether the rather schematic allocation of responsibilities, which assumes that hopeless cases were left to the practice of Asclepius, is correct (most recently HART 2000: 89). The same applies to the potency of religion in the ancient lifeworld, because this in itself can hardly explain the peaceful coexistence of the two forms either. Is it not more realistic to assume that the two seemingly divergent approaches had to be closely interlinked to allow for this kind of coexistence? SCHÄFER (2000) attempts an argument in this direction (cf. also NUTTON 1995b: 4 with note 4). A well-documented example in favour of this view is the relationship public physicians in classical Athens cultivated with the healing cults by sacrificing to Asclepius twice every year (IG II² 772). They did this not only because they felt obliged to Asclepius, but also in order to proclaim their affiliation to the medical profession (ALESHIRE 1991 and ALESHIRE 1989: 94 f.).

The fact that the methods used in the temples were not only based on the observation but also on a rational understanding of nature could be seen as another example of this interrelation. This seeming disparity needs to be critically examined and on the basis of this examination I will propose that the medicine practised within the temple precincts was also rational-scientific and therefore in keeping with the contemporary specialist literature. This thesis will be validated in a first step, in which we will attempt to approach the practice of Asclepius through the social function of its location (III.2). The second step will concern the patients themselves (III.3). The methods applied in the history of patients will be helpful in this attempt because they focus on the patients as active agents. (STEGER 2007, STEGER 2001, WOLFF 1998a/b and PORTER 1985a).

Although architecture and medicine are very classical topics, research has so far concentrated primarily on individuals or types. The social function and significance of space have been neglected for a long time and have only recently been recognized thanks to the impulses from architectural theory: for the first time social significance is being assigned to space, because space keeps being newly shaped in culturally significant ways through social practice (PRIOR 1992). Importance is also assigned to space in the social construction of illness (LACHMUND/STOLLBERG 1992). At the same time, anthropological, sociological and social elements are increasingly discussed in relation to pathogenesis so that social reality and illness are no longer seen as separate. AVALOS (1995: 56 ff.) implies this connection in his analysis of the role of the temple in the healing process. While it seems obvious that medical practice influences everyday medical culture, the same can be shown to be true for architecture, using the example of the Asclepieia in particular.

—

We can differentiate three forms of healthcare provision in the daily medical culture of the Roman Empire: bedside visits by physicians in the patient's home, patients seeing a physician in his consulting rooms (*iatreion, tabernae medicae, medicinae*), and institutional care (NUTTON 1999a and HARIG 1971).

In his *History of Hospitals*, RISSE (1999: 15–67) devotes a separate chapter to *pre-Christian sites of healing*, in which he discusses the Asclepieion and the valetudinarium, looking at both from below, that is, from the point of view of the patient, as well as from above, that is, from the point of view of the history of hospitals. In-patient healthcare is documented in an individual case where a patient is admitted to the physician's own residence that included his practice rooms (PLAUT. Men. 5.5.43 ff.): a physician recommends that Menaechmus should be taken to his house to be treated there for twenty days (HARIG 1971: 186 f.). Galen relates how he took a patient into his house for three days (GAL. De rat. cur. per ven. sect. 9.299 ff. K.). To my knowledge these two references are the only ones to this kind of in-patient treatment.

Evidence is also available for the well-established *valetudinaria* where slaves and soldiers received medical care on an in-patient basis (RISSE 1999: 38–56 and HARIG 1971: 188–195). LINDGREN (1978: 33 f.) proposes that the *valetudinaria* were the first hospitals, pointing out the model character they assumed over time. The interest in slaves and soldiers and in making sure there was institutional healthcare available for them is due to their respective function: soldiers were important for the expansion of the Roman Empire (ZIETHEN 1994: 186 and SHA Hadr. 10.8) and slaves were very valuable economically. Because of the political and economic importance of these two groups for the Empire, the state had great interest in making sure that they were looked after appropriately if they became ill. This kind of healthcare was institutionalized in the *valetudinarian*, the most eminent of which was on Tiber Island (SUET. Claud. 25.2) where diseased slaves were abandoned if their owners no longer cared to look after them. Once they had recovered their health, they were declared free by the Emperor Claudius (CASS. Dio. 60.29.7).

In the temples of Asclepius, the god of healing, patients also received care. A particular form of medicine was practised there. This practice is apparent not least in the architectural structure of the temple precinct, which is why we will discuss this aspect in more detail now. The range of treatments available in the medicine of Asclepius also included illnesses that were no longer accessible to conventional medical methods (GRAF 1998: 244). The rejected and unhealed, too, found an agency here that was able to help them. Nobody was sent away or excluded (KRUG 1993: 120 f.).

In evaluating the sanctuaries of Asclepius one also needs to consider, apart from their obvious religious significance, the myth that is attached to them, which has been discussed earlier (II.1 and III.1), as well as their political, economic, and social functions. To this end we need to look beyond the architecture to the social function and set-up of the temple, because both are of cultural importance: the sanctuary is the focus of myths and rites the elements of which leave a complex system of signs (BURKERT 1972: 39–45) that need to be deciphered. This means that the set-up in itself is of great importance (AVALOS 1995: 37 f. and GRAF 1992b: 159 f.); so is the temple's location. The best-known example is Corinth with its particularly favourable natural topography. The narrow stretch of land between the Peloponnese and mainland Greece, on the one hand, and the sea route through the Isthmus between the Saronic Gulf and the West, on the other, make this an ideal site strategically as well as in terms of transportation. In addition, one needs to consider the castle hill, Acrocorinth, which has always been a dominant feature although it is situated outside the city.

Our primary interest is therefore directed at the location of the Asclepieia: even in ancient times views differed on this point. Healing temples had to be in a salubrious environment, close to health-giving springs from which the invalid devotees could benefit (VITR. 1.2.7 and RISSE 1999: 22 f.). PLUTARCH (qu. R. 286d) wrote of the Asclepieia of Greece and Asia Minor that they occupied elevated positions because of their climatological benefits.

> Διὰ τί τοῦ Ἀσκληπιοῦ τὸ ἱερὸν ἔξω πόλεώς ἐστι; πότερον ὅτι τὰς ἔξω διατριβὰς ὑγιεινοτέρας ἐνόμιζον εἶναι τῶν ἐν ἄστει; καὶ γὰρ Ἕλληνες ἐν τόποις καθαροῖς καὶ ὑψηλοῖς ἐπιεικῶς ἱδρυμένα τὰ Ἀσκληπιεῖα ἔχουσιν·
>
> Why is the shrine of Asclepius outside the city? Is it that they considered life more healthful there than in the city? The Greeks, as one would expect, selected healthy and elevated sites for their Asclepieia.

The sanctuary of Cos, for instance, was built on a hill, three miles southwest of the city. Surrounded by cypresses and pine trees, this three-level terraced structure was built high up in an elevated position. The structure itself also rises up high, with three terraces leading up to the temple of Asclepius, which is situated on the upper terrace (figs. 8 and 11). Literary evidence can be found in the eulogies of Aristides, which will be discussed in greater depth below (III.5.1). Among all the other assets of the sanctuary at Pergamum he praises above all its clean and healthy surroundings and location (ARISTEID. or. 39.4).

The first exception from this rule is the shrine on Tiber Island (fig. 7): while elements of this Asclepieion coincide with those of the great sanctuaries in Greece and Asia Minor in that it has a temple, a cultic statue (OV. met. 15,654–656), columned halls (LIV. 2.5.4), a spring and a grove, in other words all the typical components of an Asclepieion (GRAF 1992b: 162), its location does not fit the picture. While there is certainly plenty of flowing water in the Tiber, there is no separate, and certainly no particularly healthy, spring. Moreover, its situation in the middle of the river Tiber does not even bear comparison with the great holy sites in Asia Minor and Greece. Tradition certainly never mentions any health-promoting aspects of the river Tiber. Nor is this sanctuary located in an advantageous climate outside the city. Plutarch also thought that the Asclepieion on Tiber Island needed to be explained. Following on from the passage cited above he proposes that the site was chosen by the God himself because the serpent chose to settle down there (PLUT. qu. R. 286d). One could also, as PLINY did (nat. 29.16), interpret the extraordinary location of this sanctuary on an island speculatively as an expression of the Roman distrust of Greek medicine. He does, however, not express any kind of superficial rejection of Greek medicine. His attitude can rather be explained with intertextual references and his own concept of nature. Another explanation could be the special significance of the island and its proximity to water (FEST. p. 98 L. and DEGRASSI 1987), or one can, like Plutarch, refer to the myth. (LIV. 2.5.1–4, DION. HAL. 5.13, PLUT. Publ. 8.1–5 and BESNIER 1902: 15–31).

Tiber Island, as Plutarch relates, was born from an extraordinary harvest. When the Romans had overthrown the Tarquinians and dedicated their family estate on the peninsula to the north of the city to Mars, they harvested the ripe corn on the fields there. Because the crop was consecrated to Mars, people did not dare to use it for themselves and decided to throw it into the river. There it settled in the shallow places, becoming gradually reinforced by sand and clay deposits which eventually formed Tiber Island. This mythological origin makes the island and the river itself a territory that is inaccessible to humans (GRAF 1992b: 166 f.). In 293 BCE the sanctuary of Asclepius was transferred from Epidaurus on the Peloponnese to a realm separate from the human world. The island, which was special due to its remoteness from human beings, was made available to Asclepius and his shrine. It was consecrated to him in 291 BCE, and here he could be worshipped far away from the hustle and bustle of ordinary life. A relief fragment on the quay wall (fig. 9 a/b), which commemorates the arrival of the cult of Asclepius on Tiber Island, shows a bust of Asclepius and a serpent. This Asclepieion is exceptional because of its island position. There were other shrines in Rome, apart from this, that were devoted to Asclepius. The reason for this is probably that the better situated citizens of Rome avoided the Tiber sanctuary and it therefore remained the refuge of the poor.

Although we know of no other sanctuaries of Asclepius that occupy an island of their own, there are some which were built outside a city, such as the great cultic centres of Greece and Asia Minor at Epidaurus, Cos and Per-

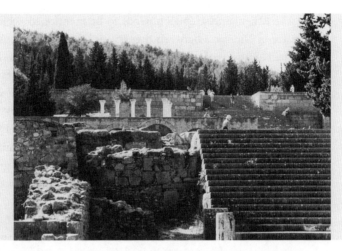

Fig. 8 –
Cos, Asclepieion:
View from the
entrance toward
the three-level
terrace

gamum. The Asclepieion at Epidaurus rises in a high valley around six miles from ancient Epidaurus. Three miles to the south-west of the ancient city of Cos lies another Asclepieion, surrounded by cypresses and pine trees. While this shrine too is on an island it does not occupy all of it. Accounts of the holy site on Tiber Island explain the difference: Cos, a busy and populated town, did not provide a precinct that was remote from human industriousness and occupation. The Pergamene Asclepieion, on the other hand, lies in a valley about three quarters of a mile to the southwest of ancient Pergamum. Pergamum, just as imperial Rome, had a dual aspect because it also had sites of worship inside the city, such as the gymnasium, for instance (OHLEMUTZ 1940: 128–130).

The Asclepian cult centres of Delos, Paros, Lebena, Epidaurus Limera, Munychia and Antium (on the latter cf. VAL. MAX. 1.8.2) are situated outside the towns, by the sea. The health-promoting properties of the Delos sanctuary are questionable, however, because although it is located outside the city it lies in a marshy bay, with a climate that is far from salubrious. The Asclepian sanctuaries of Troezen (PAUS. 2.32.4 and KRUG 1993: 145–147), Theraphne, Elis, the more recent Asclepieion at Gortys in Arcadia (JOST 1985: 205–210) and the Asclepieion of Krounoi near Naupaktos are situated across a river. Like Delos, Troezen remains a doubtful site for healing purposes despite its extra-urban situation. Even in ancient times the area around Troezen was considered to be very unhealthy (GRAF 1992b: 171) and even its elevated position on a plateau does not alter this. The older sanctuary at Gortys, the sanctuary at Aliphera, Amphissa and the Asclepieion at Aegina are situated on the slope of a steep hill (ARISTOPH. Vesp. 122 f.), as are the sanctuaries at Titani, Phlius and Patra.

Lastly, the Athenian Asclepieion needs to be mentioned, which rises above the theatre of Dionysus between the city and the Acropolis. Aside from the extra-urban locations of the Asclepian sanctuaries, which – as some examples illustrate – are not always wholesome, there are also a number of holy sites, at Corinth, Orchomenos and Messene, for example, which are situated inside the city, albeit not in the very centre, but on the fringes (EDELSTEIN/EDEL-STEIN 1945: II 234). The Corinthian sanctuary, for instance, is by the city wall. The Asclepieion at Messene is inside the city, in close proximity to the institutions of the political life, such as the Bouleuterion and the great hall of the imperial cult. The Asclepieion at Argos is close to the agora; those of Boiai, Sparta and Sicyon are inside the city.

The ancient sources specify that the Asclepieia needed to be in a healthful position and boast special springs for the patients to derive the greatest benefit during their stay (STEGER 2005b). Analysis of the position of the sanctuaries reveals that many of them are outside a city and meet these requirements, including the presence of springs (Epidaurus, Cos, and Pergamum). The unusual position of the sanctuary on Tiber Island has been discussed earlier. The investigation also shows that in some cases (Delos and Troezen) no beneficial health effects could be expected despite their extra-urban situation. And finally, there are also Asclepieia that are situated within cities.

While the location of the Asclepieia was at the centre of the first stage of our investigation, the next step is to look at the facilities themselves (SCHÄFER 2000: 262 ff. and AVALOS 1995: 47–55). Our further analysis will focus on the sanctuaries of Epidaurus (fig. 11) and Cos (fig. 12), because their architecture was the model for the later ones (COARELLI 1981: 7 f.). It is divided into the stages through which the supplicants passed as part of the healing procedure (KRUG 1993: 130–134). Ancient visitors to the Epidaurian shrine arrived at the Asclepieion from the north, from Argos or Epidaurus. The modern-day visitor takes the road from Nauplia, entering the sanctuary from the south. When the devotees arrived in this place of healing, they usually looked back on a strenuous journey and were in need of accommodation for the duration of their treatment, which might be several months. The sites therefore boasted purpose-built houses where the devotees were put up. One account survives from Epidaurus which speaks of a stay of four months (HERZOG 1931: 32). Aeschines, the orator, spent three months at Epidaurus where he was treated for a head injury (ANTH. PAL. 6.330). Aelius Aristides, of course, mentions his own two-year sojourn at Pergamum and speaks of his 'redeemer', Asclepius, whose practice/method it was to place before the eyes of the severely ill an ideal image of their life. This would stimulate the patients' creativity to overcome all hindrances posed by their illness (SCHRÖDER 1988 and III.3). These specially equipped houses were probably comparable to guest houses. PAUSANIAS (2.27.6 and 10.32.12) speaks of hostels where patients and priests resided for the duration of their stay. The sanctuaries included houses that could accommodate the devotees as well as their accompanying family members: at Epidaurus the devotees stayed to the north-west of the famous theatre in the great Xenon which boasted 160 rooms on two levels (TOMLINSON 1983: 31 ff.). The generously built hostel offered plenty of space for devotees and visitors. It included four inner courtyards which were surrounded by colonnades and by the rooms. In addition, the Epidaurian sanctuary had more houses where the administrators lived but where guests could certainly also be accommodated. In the Asclepieion at Gortys in Arcadia the temple was surrounded by numerous living quarters. At Cos (fig. 12), the lower of the three terraces offered patient accommodation. Once visitors had passed through the propylon they reached the lower level which was framed by colonnades on three sides, with long buildings extending behind them. Additional residential buildings could be found below the first terrace outside the actual sanctuary. Bathhouses have also been preserved (figs. 15 and 16). More living quarters were situated on the upper terrace. On the terraces, the middle one in particular, numerous votive offerings were displayed. The splendid three-level structure expanded along the hillside that slopes down toward the sea (fig. 17) and was erected over several generations.

Of the sanctuary at Pergamum (figs. 13 a/b) we know that the increasing number of patients made it necessary to add a new two-level healing centre in the second century CE. This extension was erected in the south-east of the complex and was linked to the older parts by a cryptoporticus. At Troezen a number of buildings were probably designated hostels. They were living quarters for patients and were not directly connected with the health treatment as such. Living and treatment quarters were strictly separated, a fact that confirms the view that the Asclepian sanctuaries cannot be seen as the first hospitals (NUTTON 1999a and KRUG 1993: 207). This is particularly obvious at Cos, where well-equipped residential buildings were situated outside the terrace building (figs. 15 and 16).

Treatments took place within the sacred precinct which consisted of the Temple of Asclepius, the altar and the abaton. At Epidaurus the sacred precinct was made up of a number of buildings which were grouped around the temple (fig. 11). Here, patients received treatment for a fixed period of time, as in a polyclinic, until they were ready to return to the guesthouses. The cult personnel were also involved in the treatment (KRUG 1993: 139), which con-

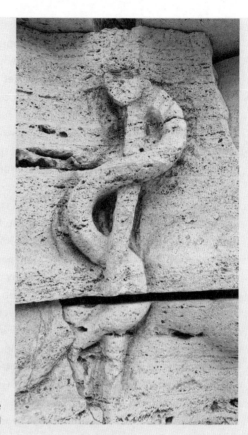

Fig. 9 a/b – Relief fragment on the quay wall of Tiber Island

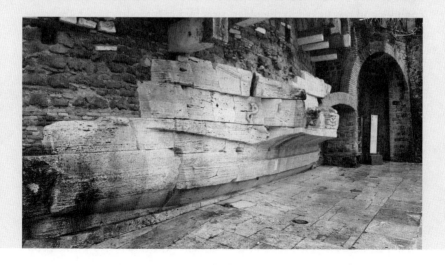

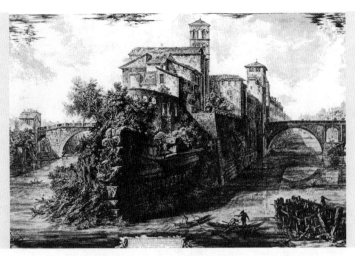

Fig. 10 –
Tiber Island
by Giovanni
Battista
Prianesi,
ca. 1780

sisted in incubation, a cultic ritual typical of the Asclepieia (HARRISSON 2014 and GRAF 1998: 246). Apart from many other healing cults (the Amphiareion of Oropus, for instance), incubation rites are also attested for the cult of Isis.

Within the sanctuary, the grove was the place where direct communication occurred between the patient and the deity, as is apparent also from the proximity of Asclepius to the oracles of Apollo at Didyma, Claros and Gryneion, which all have a grove and a spring (GRAF 1992b: 196). The grove is next to the grotto which often included a spring, as we will discuss in more detail below. At Pergamum an old plane tree grew next to the ancient spring (ARISTEID. or. 39.6), and we can assume that the sanctuary of Asclepius on Tiber Island also had a grove. A medallion of Antonius Pius shows a tree rising from the Asclepieion (BESNIER 1902: 176 fig. 19). Groves are also attested for the Asclepieia of Epidaurus (PAUS. 2.27.17), Cos (LSCG 150 A.), Gortys (CIC. nat. deor. 3.57), Titane (PAUS. 2.11.5), Epidaurus Limera (PAUS. 3.23.7), Antium (VAL. MAX. 1.8.2), Athens (IG II² 1460.28), and Kyparissia (PAUS. 4.36.7). The sacred grove of Epidaurus was home to several temples: the temple of Artemis, the statue of Epione, a shared shrine of Aphrodite and Themis (PAUS. 2.75.5) and lastly, in the northeast of the whole complex, the temple of Asclepius (TOMLINSON 1983: 57f. fig. 9f.). At Pergamum epigrams and votive offerings have been preserved which prove that, apart from Asclepius himself, members of his family were worshipped there also, including Epione, Hygieia, Panacea, Machaon and Telesphorus. But other deities, such as Artemis, Demeter and Apollo were also revered in the sanctuary of Pergamum (KRUG 1993:

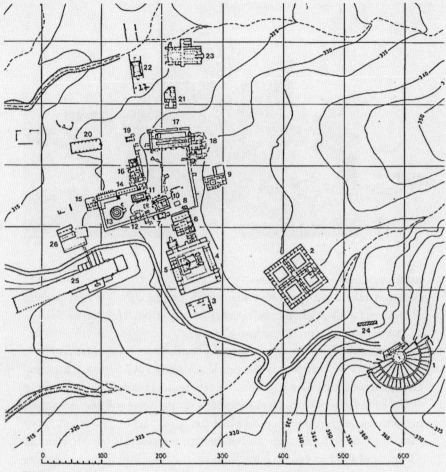

Key:

1. Theatre
2. Guest houses
3. Baths
4. Gymnasium
5. Odeion
6. Palaestra and Stoa of Kotys
7. Temple of Artemis
8. Temple of Themis
9. Temple of Asclepius and the Egyptian Apollo
10. Priest residences
11. Temple of Asclepius
12. Buildings
13. Tholos
14. Sleeping ward
15. Fountain building
16. Thermal baths and library
17. Building with Stoa
18. Thermal baths
19. Temple of Aphrodite
20. Cistern
21. Villa
22. Propylaea
23. Christian basilica
24. Museum
25. Stadium
26. Building, residence of athletes, and palaestra
27. Fountain buildings

Fig. 11 – Epidaurus, plan of Asclepieion

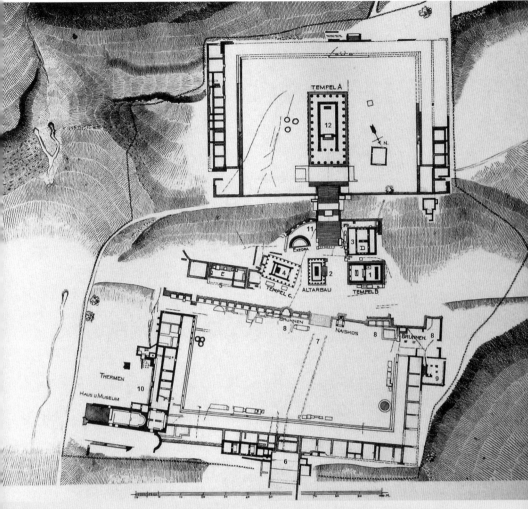

Key:

1. Ionic antae temple: temple of Asclepius
2. Altar
3. Storage for cultic objects
4. Corinthian temple of Apollo
5. Storage for votive offerings
6. Stairs to lower terrace
7. Stairs to middle terrace
8. Fountain
9. Latrines
10. Thermal baths
11. Stairs to upper terrace
12. Doric temple of Asclepius

Fig. 12 – Cos, plan of Asclepieion

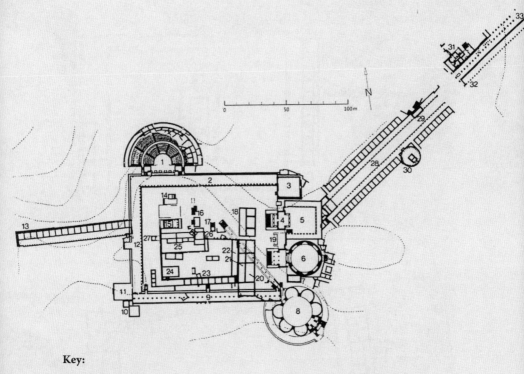

Key:

1. Theatre
2. North gallery
3. Library
4. Propylaea
5. Vestibule
6. Temple of Zeus-Asclepius
7. Cistern
8. Treatment centre (upper floor)
9. South gallery undercroft
10. Latrines
11. West gallery room
12. West gallery
13. Hellenistic Long Gallery
14. Bathing pool
15. Temple of Asclepius
16. Altars
17. Drinking pool
18. North-eastern building
19. Niche for worship
20. Eastern courtyards
21. Older Hellenistic east gallery
22. Younger Hellenistic east gallery
23. Hellenistic south gallery
24. Roman Temple
25. Incubation buildings
26. Old building
27. Rocky pool
28. Colonnaded avenue
29. Road fountain
30. Heroon
31. Thermal baths
32. Early Roman gallery
33. Via Tecta

Fig. 13 a – Pergamum, plan of Asclepieion

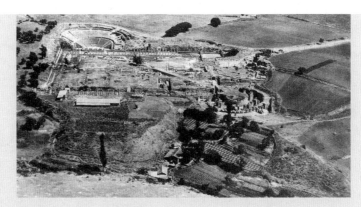

Fig. 13 b –
Pergamum,
Panoramic
view from
the South

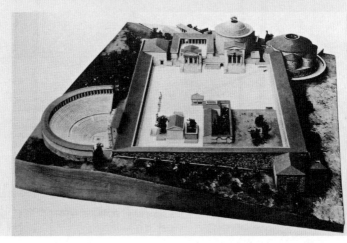

Fig. 14 a –
Pergamum,
model of
Roman
building
stage (from
the west)

165). At Cos, a temple of Apollo built in the Ionic style stood on the middle
terrace (fig. 17, on the left).

At Cos, Asclepius was also able to build on a healing cult of Apollo (SHER-
WIN-WHITE 1978: 346 f.). At Corinth, a cult is only attested for the closer family,
including aside from Asclepius only Hygieia and Podalirius, and – not least –
Apollo, whom Asclepius succeeded (LANG 1977). At Epidaurus, the devotees
arrived at an open square in front of the temple from where they could view
the precinct. The sacred complex at Epidaurus (fig. 11) has a temple from the
early fourth century BCE. This is where the famous sculpture of Asclepius
stood, which was created by Thrasymedes of Paros. An abaton, which served
as a sleeping room, formed the northern boundary of the grove. PAUSANIAS
(2.27.2) describes the cultic image in some depth. A copy of it is reproduced
in Iakovidis (1985: 19 f.), depicting Asclepius the god on a throne, with a serpent curled up beneath him (National Museum Athens No. 173, 1330, 1338 f.).

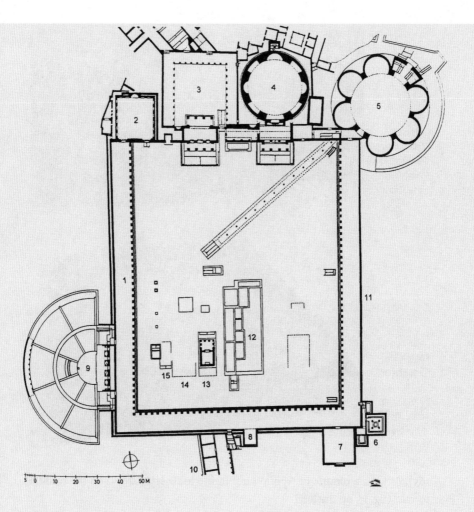

Key:

1. North gallery
2. Library
3. New propylon
4. New main temple
5. Lower round building:
   treatment centre
6. Latrines
7. West gallery

8. Exedra
9. Theatre
10. Avenue
11. South gallery
12. Incubation buildings
13. Well
14. Well
15. Old temple

Fig. 14 b – Pergamum, plan of the Roman building phase (from the west)

A long altar stood in front of the temple. In the grove there were also stelae, which listed the names of the devotees and their afflictions (PAUS. 2.27.3 f.). Early twentieth century archaeological excavations unearthed these accounts of the miraculous cures that were achieved in the Asclepieion. The stelae date back to the second half of the fourth century BCE (Herzog 1931) and provide information on the medicine practsed as part of the cult (SCHNALKE/WITTERN 1993: 99 f.). Behind the temple stood the peripteral *tholos*. This extravagant cult complex is unique because of the labyrinth in its lower part, and its mysterious shape has been much discussed by scholars (RIETHMÜLLER 1996 and ROBERT 1939). PAUSANIAS (2.27.3) speaks of a οἴκημα περιφερές. The tholos was erected during the period when major extensions were added to the sanctuary in the fourth century BCE. An inscription on the building refers to it as *thymele* (RIETHMÜLLER 1996: 72 with note 3). The tholos served as a cultic building, a heroon, and stands next to the temple that is consecrated to a god (also topographically).

One detail is important in this context: the fact that the metope decoration includes egg-shaped phials places it into a sepulchral-heroic context. Egg-shaped phials played an important part in sepulchral-heroic rites because they symbolize life, death, rebirth, but also nourishment for the dead (RIETHMÜLLER 1996: 102 with note 113). Note that in fig. 5 Asclepius is holding an egg in his right hand, which the serpent is approaching. The egg refers to the heroic cult: Asclepius was, after all, a hero first (III.1). The labyrinth can be seen as the actual cultic site for the heroic sacrifices of blood and eggs. The fact that the *tholos* building is situated at the centre of the *temenos*, and that it bears attributes associated with the hero and death cult, reveals that the site was dedicated to hero worship as well as to the worship of Asclepius.

At Cos, another Doric temple graced the upper terrace. It was situated on the central axis of the complex (figs. 18 and 19) and is reminiscent of the temple at Epidaurus, but was even bigger and more splendidly equipped (KRUG 1993: 162). Finally, a small staircase led from the upper terrace further up into a pine grove. In the cult, the temple on the upper terrace was subordinated to the temple of Asclepius with its altar on the middle terrace. Today, the remains of a Christian altar can be seen here. It was a shrine of statues and at the same time the main site of Asclepius' activity. At Pergamum, the core of the sanctuary was situated on the brow of a rock and included two temple complexes. In front of these temples were also altars. Hardly anything is left of a third temple that is said to have stood to the south, on an elevated cliff top.

Not far from the holy precinct were baths where the devotees washed before entering the temple. At Epidaurus they passed a fountain and a small

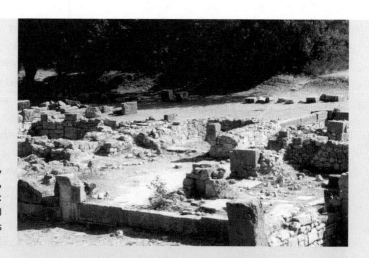

Fig. 15 – Cos, Asclepieion, entrance: residential buildings

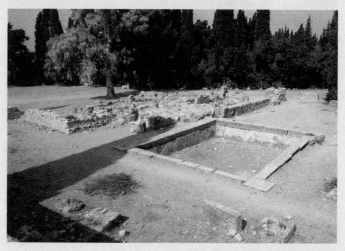

Fig. 16 – Cos, Asclepieion, entrance: residential buildings and bath

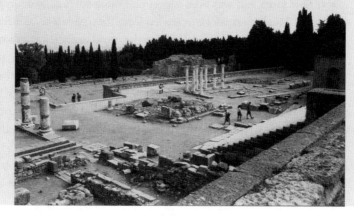

Fig. 17 – Cos, Asclepieion, view from the intermediate level (between middle and upper terrace) to the middle and lower terrace

temple, where one of the many deities besides Asclepius was worshipped, and then entered the main temple. At Pergamum the visitor, upon passing through the propylaea, stood directly in front of the temple complex with the holy spring. From there he could see the fountain buildings with the springs. Aelius Aristides describes the Hellenistic well and assigns a certain healing power to the water (ARISTEID. or. 39.6, hier. log. 2.71 and STEGER 2005b). At Cos, there were baths on the lower terrace, close to the mountain. They were incorporated in the colonnades of the wall that supported the middle terrace. The springs feeding the pools were probably rich in iron and Sulphur. On the south coast at Embros Thermae (eight miles away) hot sulphurous springs exist to this day, with rivulets running into the sea; and there are remains of ancient thermal baths on the beach at Agios Fokas. A beautiful fountain, which receives its water from Pan, has been preserved toward the left. On the lower terrace, more thermal baths remain from the second century CE. Cleaning oneself before entering the holy site was an essential component of the incubation ritual. Visitors to the Epidaurian complex entered through the propylaea, which formed the only boundary of the complex. It had no other outer walls, only boundary stones marking the site. An inscription on the propylaea reminded the devotees that anyone entering the fragrant temple had to be clean, and being clean also meant having holy thoughts (PORPH. 2.19). In Corinth, similarly, visitors entered through a simple gateway to reach the part of the complex that contained the cult buildings. At Cos the gradual purification is reflected in the terraced structure because devotees needed to climb the stairs before they reached the holy site. The complex at Troezen, like those at Corinth and Athens, has two parts, one consisting of the cultic area, the other of buildings for mundane purposes. Immediately upon entering, devotees embarked on the purification process by washing in a pool which was covered by a protective roof (AVALOS 1995: 75–78 and KRUG 1993: 141–143). The demand for purity also extended to the avoidance of actions which were not consistent with the sacredness of the site: birth and death, both extreme situations in human life, had no place inside the sanctuary. There is evidence that devotees were not permitted to give birth or die in the shrine of Delos (PARKER 1983: 33 f.). At Epidaurus, the Stoa of Kotys was erected on the edge of the holy precinct in the third century BCE. A long gallery provided space for groups who were ostracized because they were impure (PAUS. 2.27.6). In Roman times, this structure was extended by a larger bathing complex, which shows that there, too, the requirements of cleanliness and purity were observed (KRUG 1993: 134). In the Greco-Roman period it was common for visitors to carry out ritual washings before entering the sanctuary (VITR. 1.2.7 and GRAF 1992b:

179), an aspect that is particularly important in the Eleusinian sanctuaries or in the Asclepieia (BRUIT ZAIDMAN/SCHMITT PANTEL 1994: 131–140, BURKERT 1972: 274–327 and MYLONAS 1961). This view is corroborated by a comparison of the sanctuaries of Asclepius, which confirms washing as an essential and constitutive element of the cult (GUETTEL COLE 1988: 163 and MARTIN/ METZGER 1976: 62–109). The water pointed the way to the Asclepieion. In an inscription from Crete dating back to the first century BCE (ICr I 17.21), Soarchus thanks Asclepius for showing his father, Sosus, the watery path to the temple, while he was asleep. He furthermore expresses his gratitude that Asclepius appeared to him also, recommending him to use water against his father's ageing. The baths also served for implementing any balneological therapies suggested to the patients by the god. In the Asclepieion of Gortys in Arcadia a temple was built together with a bath house (KRUG 1993:185). Cos also had its own thermal baths.

People have been aware of the healing properties of water since Homer (STEGER 2005b, KRUG 1993: 172 f. and HEINZ 1996: 2412). Asclepiades already knew about the medicinal effect of water and how to use it therapeutically in a way that was compatible with his physical medicine (CELS. artes 2.17.3). Aside from its ritual significance in washing, water became increasingly important in the Hellenistic Asclepieia because of its therapeutic qualities. In the imperial period hydrotherapy grew to be an integral part of the Asclepieia and of medical therapy (Israelowich 2015: 117–124).

Healing springs, both hot and cold, were said to have a particular effect, especially during the Gallo-Roman period from which numerous votives have been preserved. KRUG (1993: 173–179) lists individual examples of structures with healing springs which are still in use today: Badenweiler in the Black Forest, Baden-Baden, Aachen, and Hochscheid in the Hunsrück mountains (all in what is now Germany). Parts of Britanno- and Hispano-Roman healing springs have also been preserved (GONZÁLEZ SOUTELO 2014 and KRUG 1993: 180 f.). Hot mineral springs rose in Pataulia (Thrace), where an Asclepieion was built in the early imperial period. During the imperial period the erection of Asclepieia was often replaced by the furnishing of healing baths with statues of Asclepius and his family (KRUG 1993: 184). We know from the sanctuaries at Cos, Epidaurus, Troezen, and Paros that the water there was of a special quality (GINOUVÈS 1962: 360 ff.). In Cos, there are Sulphur springs some distance away from the sanctuary, in the thermal baths of Embros. We have unfortunately no more precise information on the use of balneology in the Asclepieia, but we know that health spas existed in large numbers during the Roman Empire (for detailed accounts cf. HOFFMANN 1999 and HEINZ 1996:

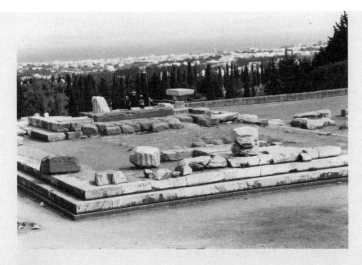

Fig. 18 – Cos, Asclepieion, upper terrace, Doric temple of Asclepius

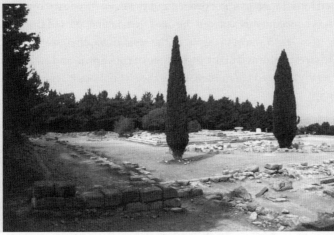

Fig. 19 – Cos, Asclepieion, upper terrace, Doric temple of Asclepius

2411 f.). Eminent among them were Vicaretto and Chiusi where the waters were considered to have a special quality (CIL XI 3294: *aquae Apollinares* and CIL XI 2092 f.). The Emperor Hadrian was said to have reserved the baths for the sick "until the eighth hour" (SHA Hadr. 22.7).

The medical view, as expressed primarily in the specialist writings of Galen, was that the bathing should follow a particular order (HEINZ 1996: 2413 f.). The accounts given by Galen and Celsus are similar: after leaving their clothes in the *apodyterium*, patients were to go on to the *tepidarium*, to warm their bodies and relax their skin (GAL. De meth. med. 10.708; 10.723 K. and CELS. artes 1.3.4). The warm bath should be briefly interrupted for the application of oil (CELS. artes 1.4.2). Then the patients should move on to the *caldarium*, where the warm, healing water was said to bring moisture to dry parts of the body. Celsus emphasized that patients should pour hot, lukewarm and then cold water on their heads (CELS. artes 1.5). The third stage of the bathing procedure took place in the *frigidarium*, where the body would cool down again, the pores close and patients be refreshed (GAL. De meth. med. 10.717 K.). Celsus does not mention the cold bath, but recommends a partial bath instead (CELS. artes 4.2.8), followed by a sweat bath. In the *sudatorium* or *laconicum* the body would release sweat. To conclude the bathing procedures the body would be rubbed with ointment. This would cause the pores to close again and replenish the skin (GAL. De meth. med. 10.481 K.). The order suggested by the physicians correlates with the architectural set-up of the baths. One often finds the sequence *apodyterium*, where patients could undress, *frigidarium* with *piscina*, *tepidarium* and *caldarium* (HEINZ 1996: 2415–2423). Sweatrooms often extended off the side of the main buildings. They need to be differentiated into the *sudatorium* proper and the dry-hot sweatroom, the *laconium*. Visitors consequently entered the *apodyterium* first, passed through the *frigidarium* in order to warm up again in the *tepidarium*, then went on to the *caldarium* to sweat, returned to the *frigidarium* to cool down, and ended by going to the laterally situated *sudatorium* where they would sweat again before the bodycare stage.

—

As part of the incubation procedure patients were also expected to present offerings after the ritual washing (BRUIT ZAIDMAN/SCHMITT PANTEL 1994: 127–130). In-depth information on the incubation ritual can be obtained from Manfred WACHT's comprehensive article in the *Reallexikon für Antike und Christentum* (1999), as well as from the fundamental writings of RENBERG (2017), SIEFERT (1980) and HAMILTON (1906), and not least also from HARRISSON (2014). Various cakes were brought for the preliminary sacrificial ritual (IG II/III² 4962 and ARISTOPH. Pl. 660 f.) and presented on a sacred table (ATHEN. 15.48.693e and IvP II 251). Next to the temple and the abaton (the sleeping hall), this sacred table was the third component of the holy precinct. We know that the middle terrace of the sanctuary at Cos boasted a large altar – still visible today – with an inner courtyard and colonnade, adorned with statues of Asclepius and the healing goddesses. Between the entrance and the temple was a long altar where sacrifices could be offered (KRUG 1993: 142 f.). This was the heart of the sanctuary. In Corinth, the sacred precinct was situated on a slightly elevated and irregular terrace. At Epidaurus, a long altar, on which offerings were presented to Asclepius, rose in front of the temple. The main offerings made to Asclepius were animals of various kinds. The sources speak of bulls (OV. met. 15.695 and IG IV² 1.41) and pigs (PHILOSTR. Ap. 1.10). Socrates, on his deathbed, asked for a cock to be sacrificed to Asclepius (PLAT. Phaid. 118a, KLOSS 2001, and MOST 1993).

The sanctuary at Pergamum specified fasting requirements: aphrodisiacs, goat's meat and cheese were not to be consumed for three days (AvP VIII.3 Nos. 161.11–14). This fasting was followed by sacrifices offered during the day to the deities Zeus Apotropaios, Zeus Meilidias, Artemis, Artemis Prothyreia, Ge and Asclepius. In the evenings, before entering the sleeping rooms, patients would offer sacrifices to Tyche, in order to obtain her favourable influence; to Mnemosyne, to make sure that they would not forget the dream; and to Themis, to ensure that the divine order would be maintained when contact was made (AHEARNE-KROLL 2014). At Epidaurus, a large building with several long galleries and colonnades stood close to the sacred precinct. The rooms, in which dining couches were found, provided a pleasant surrounding for social gatherings (TOMLINSON 1969). In Epidaurus, as in most other Asclepieia, it was not permitted to carry the sacrificed meat away: it had to be consumed onsite. The room mentioned was ideal for a large dining table where the sacrificed meat could be eaten (KRUG 1993: 134). The second part of the sanctuary at Troezen includes, in the south, a large double-span hall with three rooms furnished with dining couches. Stone tables and fireplaces provided the opportunity for sharing meals and consuming the offerings (KRUG 1993: 146).

After a ritual introduction with prayers, washings and sacrifices the patient would settle down to sleep in the temple, prepared to converse with the god. The place where he lay down is the site where the incubation would take place (IvP 264: ἐγκοιμητήριον and AvP VII.3 No. 1.4.11). Speculations abound as to this process and, compared to a rather modest amount of sources available, there is a disproportionate amount of research literature, from which the following can be derived: the sleeping halls were not accessible for anyone but the patients and cult personnel (IG IV² 1: ἄβατον is attested for Epidaurus). Patients entered this space for sleeping; it was set aside from the outside world, a highly sacred space (GRAF 1992b: 186 f.), yet despite its great importance, no architectural uniformity has been detected. At Epidaurus it was initially a *stoa,* a large room with columns on one side, a wall and a roof (GRAF 1992b: 191 f.). In the fourth century BCE an additional long hall was erected at the northern end of the sanctuary, which eventually was extended to two floors. The square building was situated on the southern edge of the sacred precinct. The modesty of the incubation room is enhanced by its situation in the stylized natural surroundings of grove and spring. At Cos, the corresponding site extended on the middle terrace, in close proximity to the altar. At Pergamum, similarly to Epidaurus, the sleeping hall was in the west of the complex (KRUG 1993: 165). In Athens, it was accommodated in a large Doric, double-span hall with an upper floor that was reached via a staircase (KRUG 1993: 150). In the sanctuary of Delos the incubation hall occupied the major part of the promontory. It was a magnificent building with an inner colonnaded courtyard (KRUG 1993: 157). Patients donned a white robe and an olive wreath before entering this area; they would wear their hair down and take off rings, belts and shoes. Once inside, they would lie down on a bed of rushes (*stibas*), which signified the connection with the outside (ARISTOPH. Plut. 663 and AvP VIII.3 No. 161.15). There is also evidence that patients were able to stretch out on an animal skin spread over a couch (LIMC II Nos 105 and 112).

From among the healing deities the appearance of the god to the patient in his sleep is most impressively documented for Asclepius (OBERHELMAN 2013 and CILLIERS/RETIEF 2013). Asclepius appears to the devotee in a dream (WALDE 2001), and either brings immediate healing or names means and ways of attaining a cure. Aside from the immediate cure during sleep, of which we learn in the reports of miracle healings (RENBERG 2017, HARRISSON 2013 and KRUG 1993: 134–141), direct healing influences also emanate from the statues, as is attested for many other gods. PAUSANIAS (9.24.3), for instance, speaks of a temple of Heracles at Hyettus, where the sick could find healing (SCHEER 2000: 87 with note 489). The dream that promises healing can also convey knowledge regarding the present and future, because in this dream a deity reveals him- or herself (OBERHELMAN 1993: 122 f.). An epigram from the Pergamene sanctuary describes how the devotee lies on his bed awaiting oneiric directions. Before lying down he had to purify himself and offer a sacrifice (HABICHT 1969: No. 161). According to the ideas expressed in the Hippocratic Corpus, on the other hand, dreams are interpreted as signs that point to underlying pathologies, usually some form of dyscrasia (HIPPOKR. Hum. 4 (5.480–482 L.), Vet. med. 10 (1.594 L.), Epid. 1.10 (2.670 L.)). Medical interpretation of dreams begins with the Hippocratic Corpus (Vict. II (6,528–291 L.) but is, beyond that, also used fruitfully in other texts, such as for instance Artemidorus' *Oneirocritica* from the second century CE (PRICE 2004, HOLOWCHAK 2001: 392 ff., and WEBER 2000). In the later tradition, Rufus of Ephesus followed the Hippocratic Corpus unreservedly (OBERHELMAN 1993: 138). Herophilus thought that there were both divine and pathophysiological causes for dreams (OBERHELMAN 1993: 135 f.). According to the empirical traditions, dreams reveal motives for actions. The Dogmatic tradition does not explicitly refer to

dreams. The Methodist tradition rejects dreams as indicators of illness (OBER-
HELMAN 1993: 136–138). Galen, finally, wrote about dreams at length, referring
to the Hippocratic tradition (GAL. In Hipp. Hum. comment. 2.2 (16.219–226
K.); In Hipp. Epid. I comment. (17.A.1–302 K.) with HOLOWCHAK 2001 and
OBERHELMAN 1993: 139–141). As a physician, he also sees dreams as possible
indicators of a pathophysiological disorder (HULSKAMP 2013). In addition,
Galen has quite differentiated ideas of the underlying meaning of a dream. In
a unique synthesis he offers a full five-point model, some aspects of which can
also be detected in other sources from the second century CE (OBERHELMAN
1993: 141 with note 95): he says that in dreams events and thoughts from the
previous day are being processed or everyday behavioural patterns repeated.
Dreams, furthermore, point to future events and they allow conclusions regarding forms of dyscrasia. The fifth criterion is the divine origin of dreams.
Speaking of the interpretation of dreams, Galen points out that they are often
difficult to understand and that telling an ordinary from a medically valuable
dream is complicated. Galen also records an oneiric healing instruction that he
himself received: when, as a youth, he suffered from chronic abdominal pain,
he dreamt he opened a vein between his thumb and index finger (GAL. De rat.
cur. per ven. sect. 9.314 f. K.). When he put this advice that he had received in
a dream into practice, his chronic pain was relieved. The dreams described by
Aristides in *Hieroi Logoi* not only convey medical information, but also refer
to the writer's importance as an eminent orator of his time. On the one hand
he compares himself in his dream with Alexander the Great (ARISTEID. hier.
log. 4.48 f.), and on the other, Plato appears to him, asking what he thought of
his, Plato's, letters as compared to Celer, the imperial official *ab epistulis* (4.57).
He points out from the very beginning that God had commended him to write
down his dreams (ARISTEID. 2.2).

The Christian church continued the tradition of incubation, replacing
Asclepius either with Christ or with a saint. The main difference was that in
Christianity the treatment was free of charge (MARKSCHIES 2006). In the
Miracula Sancti Artemii the saint appears in the dream as a physician. He
takes the patient's history and implements the therapies indicated as in an
ordinary medical consultation, following the Christian ideal (ZEPPEZAUER
2013, DÖRNEMANN 2013, and SCHULZE 2005). From the fifth to the eleventh
century, Byzantine depictions of incubations emerge in the entire Christian
territory, but primarily in Constantinople (PRATSCH 2013). While the early
Christian texts do not yet specify a distinct cultic practice, the healing sleep
was adopted as the cultic sites were Christianized. Occasionally procedures
with a medical effect were also used (herbal oils, purification, fasting, personal

caregiving, resting). The main element, however, was the trust in the god's healing power.

The importance of dreams in healing was, lastly, also transmitted to the Islamic world. Nishapur, which is situated to the east of Tehran in what is now Iran, was one of the most important translation centres of the Abbasid Caliphate. It was operated by Nestorians and specialized in the translation of Greek scientific literature. The scholar and physician Abū Al-Faraj ʿAlī ibn al-Husayn ibn Hindū from Rey, the ancient city centre of Tehran, grew up in Nishapur, where he encountered Greek science. Among other works, he composed a 'key to medicine' (*Miftah at-tibb)*, which deals mainly with the theoretical foundations of medicine, divided into accidental observations, intentional experiments, analogy to curative methods for animals, and dreams (Strohmaier 1996: 165–168).

During the incubation, the encounter with Asclepius evolved in a three-stage process, or rite of passage (VAN GENNEP 1909): in the first phase, called the separation phase, the devotee becomes detached from his everyday life and alienated from his social environment. This phase includes the ritual preliminaries, the entering into the incubation room with the appropriate rituals (white robe, olive crown) and lying down on the pallet to sleep. The second phase is the threshold- or transformation phase. During this phase the patient is put into a state of disorientation, also referred to as the "liminality phase", where he has alien, new, and sometimes disconcerting experiences. In his definition of the ritual, GEERTZ (1999: 78) describes this state as the moment when the lived and the imagined world coincide, a state when symbolic forms merge and cause the curious changes in the way reality is perceived. This is the heart of the incubation process, the encounter with the god, when – at least in the dream – the incubant has direct contact with the god (ARISTOPH. Pl. 696–763). The god grants immediate healing, speaks to him, gives advice and prescribes cures. The patient is directly confronted with the deity, in a state of total detachment from his social context (GRAF 1992b: 191). In the incubation ward the patients become >hiketai<, or supplicants (PAUS. 2.72.2 and 10.32.12), who are remote from their familiar social order and who humble themselves in the process they undergo (GOULD 1973). In the third and final phase, the phase of reintegration and incorporation, the patient, who is now transformed after meeting the deity, is reaccepted into society with his new status. Outwardly, this reintegration is marked by the patient's removing the olive crown and placing it on the pallet (*stibas*). A shared meal follows during which the sacrificial meat is being consumed (AvP VIII.3 No. 161.13 f. and GRAF 1992b: 194 f.). This concludes the incubation process and the devotee is received back into his usual environment. He leaves the sacred precinct, pays an appropriate fee to the temple administration and makes a thank-offering to Asclepius. Asclepius expected adequate payment for the help he granted (KRUG 1993: 134). In Corinth there was an offering box in the sacred precinct: a hollowed-out stone into which a vessel with a slatted lid was inserted (KRUG 1993: 142). In Epidaurus the income obtained served to pay for the staff, building material and the maintenance of the sanctuary. The sums expended are attested in epigrams (RENBERG 2017: 260–268, KRUG 1993: 132 and BURFORD 1969).

The countless devotions found in the Asclepieia at Epidaurus, Cos, Pergamum and Athens reflect the gratitude, piety and trust of the visitors, but they were also advertisements that helped the sanctuaries to grow. The temple complex at Cos is a good example of this: on the right side of the sanctuary was a cultic shrine, in which the *archiatros C. Stertinius Xenophon* dedicated a statue to the Emperor Nero. The sanctuary flourished thanks to the activities and influence of Xenophon. Donations made it possible to extend the complex and install a medical library. Xenophon's efforts and influence corroborate the thesis that some Asclepieia enjoyed extraordinary privileges and that they benefited from the donations and offerings that provided material security. Without this foundation the continued care for the sick and weak would have been inconceivable.

The complexes also included theatres and stadiums for performances and contests. All these buildings were part of a holistic therapy concept. Architecture had a significant social role to play in this context and constitutes a vital aspect of the type of medicine practised in the Asclepieia.

A magnificent theatre, built in the third/second century BCE, stood on the southern edge of the temple complex at Epidaurus. PAUSANIAS (2.27.5) mentions Polycleitus the Younger as its architect (plan reproduced in PAPACHATZIS 1978: 138). The theatre, as well as the stadium in the southwest and the slightly more remote hippodrome, were built for the arts and sports contests which were held every five years as part of the festival of Asclepius (KRUG 1993: 133). It was destroyed by the Goths in 267 CE, but was reconstructed and remains famous for its striking acoustics (TOMLINSON 1983: 31–33). In the second century CE the Roman senator Antoninus Pythodorus from Nysa in Asia Minor donated a considerable sum for extensive architectural changes at the complex in Epidaurus, including thermal baths with mosaic floors and a library (TOMLINSON 1983: 31 f.). In Roman times an extensive bath complex was added. Pergamum also had a theatre in the north of the sanctuary and close-by, to the north-east, a library which consisted in a rectangular room with fitted shelves and cases for books and scrolls (KRUG 1993: 168).

The last extensive building phase at Pergamum in pre-Roman times was in the third century BCE, when the Attalids made the city their residence (RADT 1999: 220). After the destruction of the site by Seleucus IV and its reconstruction under Hadrian not much was left of the original complex (KRUG 1993: 165 f.). According to Aristides (hier. log. 4.64), countless miracle healings occurred in the Pergamene sanctuary during the reign of Domitian (PETSALIS-DIOMIDIS 2010: 37, DRÄGER 1993: 176–180, and HABICHT 1969: 6–8). Under Hadrian, the site was extensively restructured: during his first visit in Asia Minor in 123 CE the emperor commissioned new buildings, which he then inaugurated on the occasion of his second visit in 129 BCE. After experiencing a phase of decline up until the middle of the imperial period, the Asclepieion in Pergamum rose to new heights and grew to be one of the most important sanctuaries in Asia Minor and a supra-regional site of pilgrimage (RIETHMÜLLER 2011: 232, PETSALIS-DIOMIDIS 2010: 167–172, and HALFMANN 2001: 56–58). The new buildings were funded thanks to Hadrian's personal contacts among the influential and wealthy families in Pergamum. Claudius Charax financed the monumental propylaea in the north with its courtyard surrounded by colonnaded galleries (PETSALIS-DIOMIDIS 2010: 178–185 and ZIEGENAUS/DE LUCA 1981: 5–29). To the south Rufinus built the temple of Zeus Asclepius (PETSALIS-DIOMIDIS 2010: 194 and HALFMANN 2001: 56 f.). This Asclepieion was later included among the wonders of the world as the "Grove of Rufinus" (ANTHOL. GRAEC. 9,656 and PETSALIS-DIOMIDIS 2010: 194). Both Rufinus and Charax belonged to the *ordo senatorius* (senatorial elite). Flavia Melitine donated the library, Pollio paid for the north gallery, which he devoted to Asclepius, the other gods and Hadrian. He was also admitted to the senate. Unlike the Asclepieion on Tiber Island in Rome, the great sanctuaries of Greece and Asia Minor were of high repute among the wealthy Roman families. MARTIAL (9.16.2) referred to Asclepius as *Pergameus deus*, STATIUS (silv. 3.4.23 f.) as *maximus aegris auxiliator*. The Asclepieion at Pergamum became the place to meet for many of the rich and prominent citizens of the Roman Empire. With the number of visitors steadily rising, more accommodation was required. Particularly in the later period, noticeable efforts were made at most of the Asclepieia to add extensions. In the sanctuary of Cos, for instance, the need for multi-seat latrines was addressed (KRUG 1993: 162). With the growing reputation of the Asclepieia as intellectual centres, their interior assumed greater importance over their remote exterior situation (GRAF 1992b: 198 f.). Even the Emperor Caracalla visited the sanctuary in Pergamum for incubation on his Eastern campaign in the summer of 214 CE, hoping to be granted healing dreams (HERODIAN. 4.8.3 and BIRLEY 1997: 190 f.). Pergamum had become the abode of the Muses, who invited visitors for a health-bringing sojourn at this cultural and societal hub.

III.3 – The sources – mere miracle stories?

After looking at the location and social function of the Asclepieia in the previous chapter (III.2) we will now zoom in on the patients who received care in the temple complexes of Asclepius. Introspective testimonies are few and far between and those that exist do not provide much detail. Nonetheless, these reports, such as dreams recorded in conjunction with thank-offerings, need to be consulted. Some dreams are described on sacrificial dedications left by the supplicants after they received oneiric healing or prescriptions to improve their health (AVALOS 1995: 65–70, VAN STRATEN 1981 and RÜTTIMANN 1986: 36–178). These devotional offerings could be purchased by patients on their way to the sanctuary, in the street shops of Pergamum, for instance, or at the sanctuaries during their stay. Visitors arriving from Pergamum would reach the Asclepieion by the *via tecta* which then turned into a colonnaded avenue. Walls were erected between the columns to form shops trading in dedicatory gifts (RADT 1999: 227 and RÜTTIMANN 1986: 69–93). Depending on individual means, these sacrifices could be simple tablets made of wood or clay (*sanides* or *pinakes*), sculpted reproductions of the diseased body part or even marble votive reliefs and sculptures of Asclepius and his family. While it seems possible to infer the social rank of a dedicant from such votive gifts, this proves more difficult upon closer scrutiny (FORSÈN 1996: 165–168): firstly, the anatomical votives were almost uniform with hardly any detectible differences, and secondly, one can only infer within certain limits a dedicant's social status from an expensive votive offering. Researchers assume that the supplicants came from all social strata and presented with a wide range of afflictions (KOELBING 1977: 62, SCHADEWALDT 1967 and EDELSTEIN/EDELSTEIN 1945: 116 f.). This was not true, as we have seen in chapter III.1, of the Asclepieion on the Tiber Island. At Epidaurus, the dedicants were able to view earlier votive offerings after making their sacrifices in the sanctuary. Offering their own gifts had a positive psychological effect on the patients because they firmly believed that the deity would help them (SCHNALKE 1990: 28 ff.). The pagan ritual of votive-giving was later also adapted at Christian sites of pilgrimage and reached its apex during the Baroque period (KRUG 1993: 132 and 134–141).

PAUSANIAS (2.27.3) relates having seen six stelae at Epidaurus. The priests in that sanctuary encouraged patients to have stone stelae erected with reports of their healing rather than the less durable tablets made of wood. It is possible that the preserved stone inscriptions include excerpts from the votive tablets fashioned by the priests (KRUG 1993: 135). Archaeological excavations at Epidaurus unearthed seventy reports of miraculous healings mostly dating back to late on in second half of the fourth century BCE. They are on three of the six stelae mentioned and on fragments of a fourth (IG IV² 1.121–124, LIDONNICI 1995 and HERZOG 1931). Similar devotional testimonies from Cos described by STRABO (8.6.15) have not been preserved. Regarding finds from other Asclepieia before 1945 the collection of EDELSTEIN/EDELSTEIN (1945) can be consulted, as can HABICHT (1969: No. 63–144) for inscriptions discovered at the Asclepieion in Pergamum up until 1964. A number of individual investigations exist for the later years (such as PEEK 1963).

In Lebena on the southern coast of Crete visitors left tablets inscribed with reports of their healing experiences. At the behest of the priests some were carved into the back wall of the abaton (sleeping chamber) in order to preserve them, in a similar fashion to those at Epidaurus (ICr XVII 9.17–19.24 and GUARDUCCI 1934). A small altar still exists from the Asclepieion at Athens, which was well attended and replete with dedicatory and anatomical votive offerings (ALESHIRE 1989). The altar had been repurposed and was found in the wall of a residence from a later time, situated to the west of the Prytaneion (BÜYÜKKOLANCI/ENGELMANN 1991: 143 f. No. 10 with tablet 10). The story behind it tells of Zosimus, the agent of Flavia Modesta, who suffered from headaches and an eye problem. Asclepius and Hygieia healed his afflictions and out of gratitude he erected the altar to these deities. There were special halls for the storage of votive offerings. On the middle terrace at Cos the foundations of such a hall are still discernible next to the temple of Asclepius (figs. 12 and 17). Numerous votive offerings and dedicatory inscriptions have also been found at the sanctuary on Tiber Island in Rome (KRUG 1993: 164 and RÜTTIMANN 1986: 57–64).

While an abundance of gift offerings remain for Pergamum, Epidaurus and Athens, there are only indirect indications of votive gifts at other sites, such as Corinth for instance. These include above all indentations in the ground of the sanctuary's yard which indicate that there used to be columns and bases for votive offerings (KRUG 1993: 142 f.). It is therefore almost impossible to reconstruct the healing practice of Corinth. Apart from the finds mentioned there is one from the early imperial period that is particularly important for the relationship between cult and medicine: an epigraph from the Asclepieion containing a tribute to C. Vibius Euelpistus, who was a priest as well as a physician at the sanctuary. No other details remain.

The same is true for the many smaller and less significant Asclepieia that were scattered across the islands. One of them was on the island of Paros. The numerous votive reliefs and inscriptions found there suggest that this site must have been highly respected locally (KRUG 1993: 156). Similarly at the sanctuary at Delos: the fact that almost a hundred tablets were found there seems to attest to the site's great popularity (KRUG 1993: 157). Even for the provinces of Gallia and Germania donations in honour of Asclepius are documented in altogether eleven inscriptions that contain references to *Aesculapius/Asclepius* (SCHWINDEN 1994: 138 f. with note 35 f.). One inscription from a prominent patron, T. Iulius Saturninus, *procurator Augustorum*, was found in Trier (CIL XIII 3636) and dates back to the times of Emperor Marcus Aurelius and his co-ruler Lucius Verus. It was during their reign, from 166 CE onwards, that the empire was struck by a devastating plague (GILLIAM 1961, and more recently the contributions in LO CASCIO 2012). Against the backdrop of this epidemic the donation can either be interpreted as a *votum* made after the illness was overcome, or as a prophylactic gift from Iulius Saturninus, either as a private person or on behalf of the emperor. In addition to the major sanctuaries (Pergamum, Epidaurus and Cos) there were consequently, as the objects and documents that have been preserved testify, a number of smaller Asclepieia. For Cos no healing reports or votive reliefs have been found but numerous inscriptions of a religious or political nature, some of which can still be viewed today in a rudimentary museum that forms part of the complex (KRUG 1993: 163).

The devotees left donations either out of gratitude for having been healed or because they hoped to be relieved from an affliction (MARTZAVOU 2012). The tokens of gratitude were often anatomical dedications (FORSÈN 1996: 9–27 and DRAYCOTT/GRAHAM 2017). The fact that more than a third of all anatomical votives from the Aegean region depicting body parts were found in Asclepian sanctuaries (Athens, Piraeus, Corinth, Eleusis, Epidaurus, and Pergamum) confirms the eminent position Asclepius occupied among the healing deities (FORSÈN 1996: 145). Anatomical votives were also discovered in the Asclepieia of Cos, Delos, Crete, Paros, Messene, Thessaly, and Macedonia (FORSÈN 1996: 2–4). The three-dimensional votive gifts contain images of almost all parts of the human anatomy, but rarely internal organs (DRAYCOTT/GRAHAM 2017). Research into the sources commonly suggests that little attention was given to pathological changes which might yield information on the distribution of illnesses.

A well-preserved and well-known anatomcal votive from Epidaurus is of two ears (National Musem Athens 1428 and FORSÈN 1996: No. 13.1 with note

83) carved opposite each other into a square marble relief. The dedicatory inscription below these ears is from the first century CE and confirms Cutius Gallus as the dedicant and his ears as the organs affected by illness. The epigram indicates that Cutius was healed from this affliction (IG IV² 1.440). Similar depictions of ears were also found in Corinth (fifth/fourth century BCE) (KRUG 1993: 144 f.). They symbolize the hope expressed by the dedicant that the god may grant an ear to the dedicant's prayer. Most of the thank-offerings in Corinth suggest gynaecological disorders, while those in Epidaurus point to ocular diseases (CHANIOTIS 1995: 329 and HERZOG 1931: 95–97). A votive from the second century CE, found in the Asclepieion at Athens, depicts a male behind, from the waist down to the hollow of the knees. What is left of the inscription mentions the dedicant, Lykos, who installed this votive gift to Asclepius (IG II² 4518). From the Asclepieion at Melos votives in the form of a left foot and a left ear are documented (Epigraphical Museum Athens 3224 and FORSÈN 1996: No. 33.2 with fig. 113). The square marble relief shows a left lower leg up to the knee, with the foot turned to the left. To the right of the foot one sees a left ear and to the left a dedicatory inscription to Hygieia and Asclepius which can be dated to the Hellenistic or Roman period. The name of the dedicant has not survived (IG XII 3.1087). From the Asclepieion on Tiber Island numerous terracotta votives have been preserved, all depicting healed organs. They were discovered between 1881 and 1890 when major works were carried out on the Tiber river (PENSABENE/RIZZO/ROGHI/TALAMO 1980).

Some of these devotional offerings document immediate miraculous cures reminiscent of the Christian miracle reports (SCHADEWALDT 1967: 1756 and WEINREICH 1909). Reports of faith healings have been transmitted by Augustine, for instance (AUG. civ. 22.8 and GÜNTHER 2000: 263), who obviously strove to strengthen the faith of his readers. They are, however, characterized by their proximity to magic rather than faith. Miracle cures are also known from the Asclepieia: eminent among these are the cures achieved by Asclepius at Epidaurus, of which we learn from PAUSANIAS (2.27.3), and from four surviving stelae (IG IV² 1.121–124) (LIDONNICI 1995 and LIDON-NICI 1992: 25 with note 5). The altogether seventy dedications reflect a wide demographic and geographical breadth (SOLIN 2013). KRUG (1993: 134–141) cites several examples from the Iamata and, building on HERZOG (1931), adds psychological and psychosomatic aspects to his interpretation, which he underpins with archaeological evidence. Persons of all ages, from individuals to families with children, prayed to Asclepius that he might heal their illnesses. Of the 48 detailed Epidaurian healing reports 31 are from men, 13 from women and four from children (DILLON 1994: 245). It has been pointed out that the collection emerged gradually and that it is part of a longer tradition. While LIDONNICI (1995) emphasizes the psychological effect of the votive offerings as an expression of belief and hope, HERZOG (1931) reads them as medical sources. The historicity of these miraculous cures, whether or not they have a medical component, is called into question. SOLIN (2013) recently denied any connection between the dream cult and medicine. EDELSTEIN/EDELSTEIN (1945) and MEIER (1967) emphasize the experiential nature of the sources. They are documented reflections of individuals and provide insight into the faith people had in Asclepius (DILLON 1994: 253 with note 74). RÜTTIMANN (1986: 44–57) focused on the Epidaurian testimonies from the perspective of the second century CE, evaluating them primarily from a religious-historical point of view. HARRISSON (2013) examined dream reports in the historical and fictitional literature from the Roman Imperial period.

During the third century BCE, miraculous healings (*Iamatica*) were also described by the epigrammatist Poseidippus. Poseidippus spent much of his life at the court in Alexandria, where euergetic foundations took care of cults, shrines and the arts. Poseidippus was, next to Callimachos, an important Ptolemaic court poet. He wrote these *Iamatica* in a poetic form, which means that the suffering is formally presented in long passages, whereas the healing is depicted in a short form; in other words, the content is poetically exaggerated. This papyrus, published in 2001, contains seven epigrams consisting of 32 verses which are dealing with Iamatika (95–100; MÄNNLEIN-ROBERT 2015: 343–374) and represent a collection of healing stories from an unknown sanctuary of Asclepius.

These healing stories again provide names, some of them also the origins and illness of the individuals mentioned. They are set in the sacred area, the *Temenos* of an Asclepieion. Epigram 95 is an exception in that its location is the Delphic sanctuary of Apollo. An important question remains, however, and that is whether these are historical documents or poetic creations. There is some evidence that Poseidippus, in playing with the conventions of established epigraphy creates a literary genre. This means that a purely Hellenic sacred sphere is deliberately conjured up here with references to Hellenic divinities such as Apollo and Asclepius. The epigrams testify to spontaneous healings of hopeless cases through the art of medicine, which are performed at the last moment (95), take place during a sacrifice for Asclepius (96), occur after sleep in the temple (97, 98, 100) or after the prayer to Asclepius (99). They describe a possible course of events in an Asclepieion. At the same time, they attest to a Panhellenic expansion of the cult, to Delphi (95), Cos (97) and Lebena on Crete (99). Snakebite, paralysis, epilepsy, infection, deafness and blindness are the typical medical conditions described. The Iamata of Epidaurus served as a template for this (IG IV² 1.121–124), with noticeable, strong references to the miraculous cures (121 and 122). Poseidippus' *Iamatica* provide an example of a purposely arranged group of epigrams that focus on miraculous and rapid healings. With the exception of epigram 96, these epigrams, which are composed in distichs, are short and devoid of passages devoted to the praise of a deity.

πρὸς σὲ μὲν Ἀντιχάρης, Ἀσκληπιέ, σὺν δυσὶ βάκτροις
ἦλθε δι' ἀτραπιτῶν ἴχνος ἐφεκλόμενος
σοὶ δ[ὲ θυη]πολέων εἰς ἀμφοτέρο[υ]ς πόδας ἔστη
καὶ τὸ π[ο]λυχρόνιον δέμνιον ἐξέφυγε.

To you, Asclepius, came Antichares, on two crutches
as he traced a trail on the way;
he sacrificed to you and stood on his feet,
and he escaped the bed he was tied to for a long time. (96)

Epigram 96 refers to the sudden healing of the footsore Antichares during a sacrifice to Asclepius. With a few exceptions the text is well preserved and expresses the great gratitude of the healed man. Whether it was a miraculous cure, as the literature claims, is questionable (MÄNNLEIN-ROBERT 2015).

The *Iamatica* imitate genuine inscriptions but are in fact short literary epigrams, which focus on the transition from sickness to health and include the names of the persons speaking. This explains the absence of the Doric dialect present in the *Iamata*. Poseidippus' *Iamatica* are a new genre that includes a purposeful collection of selected texts composed as a cycle that can be read as serious or ironic. The reader in this case is confronted with epigrams of a sacred context on papyrus scrolls and therefore clearly in a different situation – in terms of space and time – from the reader in an Asclepieion.

οἷος ὁ χάλκεος οὗτος ἐπ' ὀστέα λεπτὸν ἀνέλκων
πνεῦμα μόγι[ς] ζωὴν ὄμματι συλλέγεται,
ἐκ νούσων ἐσάου τοίους ὁ τὰ δεινὰ Λιβύσσης
δήγματα φαρμάσσειν ἀσπίδος εὑρόμενος
Μήδειος Λάμπονος Ὀλύνθιος, ὧι πανάκειαν
τὴν Ἀσκληπιαδῶν πᾶσαν ἔδοκε πατήρ·
σοὶ δ', ὦ Πύθι' Ἄπολλον, ἑῆς γνωρίσματα τέχνης
λείψανον ἀνθτρόπου τόνδ' ἔθετο σκελετόν.

As this bronze statue is emaciated to the bones,
hardly breathes, and collects life in his view,
from these diseases the same person rescued patients, who against terrible bites
of the Libyan adder a remedy he found
Medeius, son of Lampon, from Olynth, to whom the universal remedies
of the Asclepiads handed over the father;
for you, Apollo from Pytho, as proof for his art
as last thing he erected this sceleton, what remains of man. (95)

Poseidippus' proximity to the Ptolemaic royal court is also attested by epigram 95, a votive epigram by the physician Medeios: He consecrates a bronze statue to Apollo, which is to be erected in Apollo's sanctuary in Delphi. In this case, a seriously ill person in a cachectic state is described who, reduced to a skeleton after a snakebite, is rescued by Medeios. The text which, apart from a few letters, is well preserved, contains some spelling mistakes and is written in the Attic-Ionian dialect. The literature on the topic refers to this text as an example of a miraculous healing (MÄNNLEIN-ROBERT 2015), a view that is difficult to understand given that the cure is performed by a physician who treats a snakebite with a remedy for poisoning. The medical procedure rather provides a further argument in favor of an independent medicine of Asclepius. The fact that Medeios brings a nearly doomed person back to life is, however, reminiscent of the well-known Asclepian motif. It should also be noted that it is not a dedication to Asclepius but to Apollo, although the proximity between the two is close. This aspect, too, is only superficially discussed in the relevant literature.

ὄλβον ἄριστος ἀν[ηρ], Ἀσκληπιέ, μέτριον αἰτεῖ
– σοὶ δ᾽ ὀρέγειν πολλὴ βουλομένωι δύναμις –
αἰτεῖται δ᾽ ὑγιείαν, ἄκη δύο· ταῦτα γὰρ εἶναι
ἠθέων ὑψηλὴ φαίνεται ἀκρόπολις.
Moderate wealth, Asclepius, the best man demands
– for you, it is easily possible to grant it –,
for himself he demands health: two remedies; they seem
to be a proud acropolis for the morals. (101)

Epigram 101 is a supplication to Asclepius, invoking or praying for prosperity and health as the two most important means of healing or salvation. The text was corrected in two places (lines 1 and 3). In addition to healing remedies and healing sleep, wealth – or rather health – are the main therapeutic motifs. This confirms the origin of the epigram in Hellenism, a period informed by plurality with religious healing in the sense of miracle cures on the one hand, and rational healing on the other. This tension between a sense of obligation toward the gods and human merit based on *techne* is also evident in the framing epigrams. Epigram 101 could consequently also be addressed to the physician Medeios and be variously interpreted as irony, skepticism or humor.

These epigrams were created by a *poeta doctus*. Poseidippus may have presented a commissioned work here – a literary narrative interspersed with ironic moments. On the surface, the text may be concerned with medical and religious remedies, but they are in fact literary-poetic remedies against popular and religious superstition.

As we return to epigraphic sources, there are several other inscriptions citing miracle healings over and above the Epidaurian Iamata. An inscription from 224 CE records how Tiberius Claudius Severus of Sinope was instructed in a dream (κατ᾽ ὄναρ) to leave this testimony to Asclepius, his *soter* (σωτῆρι Ἀσκληπιῷ) and to Apollo Maleatas, on whose cult Asclepius was able to build in Epidaurus (IG IV² 127 and RÜTTIMANN 1986: 48 f.). The God appeared to him in the *enkoimeterion* and took away the illness that had affected his throat and ears. Diophantus of Sphettus, who, according to his own words, could not expect help from any mortal and who believed that only Asclepius had the power to cure him, left an inscription to Asclepius in Athens (IG II² 4514 from the second century CE). He turned to Asclepius asking for relief from the pain in his feet (ποδάγρα), because, as a temple servant, he wished to be able to enter the house of Asclepius as cheerfully as before – and he was cured. An inscription from the second century found in Rome renders the questionable character of these reports more apparent (IG XIV 966 with RÜTTIMANN 1986: 58 f.). It narrates four miraculous healings of men who could not find help anywhere else (ἀφηλπισμένοι): 1. A blind man called Gaius was instructed by Asclepius to approach the altar in a reverent attitude, bow to the god, then walk around the altar from right to left, place his five fingers on the altar, remove his hand again and place it on his own eyes. Suddenly he could see again. 2. Lucius, who had suffered from a pain in his side (πλευρειτικός), was told by Asclepius to approach the altar, gather the ashes there, mix them with wine and paste the mixture on his side. He also was immediately released from his affliction. 3. Julian kept bringing up blood. Asclepius ordered him to collect pine nuts at the altar and eat them three days in a row with honey. He was also cured. 4. Finally, Asclepius ordered Valerius Aper, a blind soldier, to take the blood of a white cock, mix it with honey and apply the salve to his eyes. He was also cured. Blindness and the regaining of vision are frequent topics. They are also mentioned in an inscription from Crete (third century CE), in which Diodorus dedicates two statues to the dream healer Asclepius in gratitude for having his vision restored (ICr I 17.24).

Miracle healings did not only occur in the Asclepieia. They are also documented in connection with the emperors Vespasian and Hadrian (WEBER 2000: 382–388, CLAUSS 1999: 113–115, 346 f., and HAEHLING VON LANZENAUER 1996: 59–91). One of the main tasks of emperors was to ensure the wellbeing of the state (ZIETHEN 1994: 171 f. and 178–181). Actions performed by emperors with a view to eliminating public grievances were often described in biological terms, because the state was seen as a living organism (LIV. 2.32.8–12). Considering the expectations people had of their emperor, it is understandable that he was seen as a therapist and soter: the emperor takes on the role of a healer (ZIETHEN 1994: 176 with notes 23–25). When emperors met the delegates from the provinces or cities or when they visited the provinces and cities, they tended to make every effort to establish harmonious and stable relationships, and miracle healings were part of this process. In November 69 CE Vespasian travelled to Egypt (MORENZ 1949/50) and during his stay there he performed healings of the sick. He used these, his first actions in office, as propaganda and means of self-presentation throughout the empire (TAC. hist. 4.81). As the emperor he had to ensure the wellbeing of the citizens and, particularly in the eastern part of the empire, he had to live up to the traditional expectation of the emperor acting as Saviour (ZIETHEN 1994: 181 with note 58). He therefore betook himself to the Serapeum in order to ask the Oracle about his future as an emperor. From there he went on to the Hippodrome where he received the acclamations of the people (P. FUAD 1.8 and MONTEVECCHI 1981). Two men, one blind (*tabes oculorum*) and the other with a crippled hand (aeger manum), approached the emperor after dreaming of Serapis had encouraged them to declare themselves to the ruler, and besought healing from Vespasian. In contrast to the healings performed by Asclepius or to the Christian faith healings, the supplicants in this case expected detailed directions for them to put into practice. Vespasian was hesitant at first, but after thorough consultation with his courtiers and – more importantly – with the physicians, he gave in to the supplicants' wishes (TAC. hist. 4.81, SUET. Vesp. 7, PHILOSTR. Ap. 5.28–30, and CASS. DIO 66.8.1). He tread the crippled man's hand with his foot and wiped the eyes of the blind man with his saliva and both were miraculously healed. Saliva was considered to carry soul forces (PLIN. nat. 28.4.7 and Ziethen 1994: 184). The healing with the foot entails a reference to Serapis. Numerous votive tablets depict marble feet crowned with the head of Serapis. The same motif appears in the second century CE on Alexandrian coins (DOW/UPSON 1944).

There is also a parallel in the power of the foot of Asclepius to cure paralysis (IG IV 952 and ZIETHEN 1994: 183 with note 68).

The curative effects honoured the performer of the healing action (MORENZ 1949/50: 371). Vespasian implemented the directions of the Alexandrian Serapis and was therefore able to claim divine legitimation from the very beginning of his reign. By doing his duty in a local incident he achieved sacral legitimation (LEVICK 1999: 68 f.). Vespasian was therefore the earthly image of Serapis and at the same time an emperor blessed by the gods. He performed the act of healing as *princeps electus divinus ministerio* (TAC. hist. 4.81.2). As a *homo novus* Vespasian was unable to refer to a deified imperial ancestor (MALITZ 1997). His performing of miracles can therefore be regarded as Flavian propaganda that made him appear as *princeps legitimus* authorized by the gods. Because of their propagandistic nature the healings can also be seen as imitations of Alexander. Alexander founded Alexandria on the site of an ancient chapel dedicated to Serapis. He also went by himself to the sanctuary of Zeus Ammon at Siwa Oasis. He was often able to help his friends as a result of the medical knowledge he had acquired from his teacher Aristotle (WEBER 2000: 384 with note 111, HAEHLING VON LANZENAUER 1996: 78–80). The political significance of Vespasian's miraculous healings is evident. It is therefore the more surprising that CHRIST (1995) does not mention them in his overall presentation of the imperial period. The healing incidents brought Vespasian popularity and legitimacy in Egypt and in other eastern provinces, and equipped him perfectly for his fight against Vitellius, whom he would defeat soon afterwards.

Similar miraculous cures are also documented in connection with the Emperor Hadrian who became seriously ill after his victory over the Jews in the Bar Kokhba revolt (from 136 CE). He had suffered from nose bleeds for some time and as a result lost so much blood (CASS. DIO 69.17.1) that he seemed almost consumptive (CASS. DIO 69.20.1). In addition, he suffered from dropsy, with attacks of fever aggravating his general condition (SHA Hadr. 25.3). Although he found it difficult to endure this and repeatedly considered suicide, he was concerned that others should be healed (SHA Hadr. 25.1–4): a woman, of whom no more details are known (*quaedam mulier*) received direction in a dream to inform Hadrian that he should not take his own life, because he would recover. She did not carry out this task and became blind. The same directions were given to her in another dream, in which she was also told to kiss the emperor's knee because this would restore her eyesight. The woman now did as she was told and could see again after washing her eyes with water from the stream that ran past the sanctuary from which she had just come:

probably the Serapeum in the city of Rome or the sanctuary of Asclepius on Tiber Island. A conclusive identification is not possible. The critical evaluation of this source has been repeatedly referred to, most recently by WEBER (2000: 387 with notes 135 and 136). A comment made by SUETON (Hadr. 25.4) suggests that, according to Marius Maximus, there was some deceit involved in the miracles described, which may explain why CHRIST (1995: 328) omitted any mention of them. But even if the historicity of these events needs to be critically interrogated, the topos of the emperor as healer survives. CLAUSS (1999: 346 f.) presents Hadrian's healing of the sick as historical occurrences. The second miracle healing concerns a blind old man from Pannonia who touched Hadrian when he was sick with fever and shortly afterwards his vision was restored, while Hadrian gained a fever-free period from the encounter. Both miracle reports are connected with Hadrian's own illness. In both cases, Hadrian himself benefited from the healing of a sick person.

While reports abound of miracle healings similar to the Christian miracle reports, and while these provided propaganda in support of the image of the "emperor as healer," there is also a wealth of documented dream instructions which convey information on the therapeutic methods used to alleviate the suffering of the patients during their stay in a sanctuary. KRUG's (1993: 135) argument that the psychosomatic foundation of many of the afflictions is a generally accepted fact today that casts an explanatory light on many of the reports, must be rejected. KRUG commits the same anachronistic as well as methodical mistake that has induced many others to venture a retrospective diagnosis. But the god does not help the patients through his presence alone, but provides therapies which are in no way inferior to a stay in a health spa. These methods are less spectacular than is sometimes assumed and those presented as spectacular belong to the domain of the miracle reports. EDEL-STEIN/EDELSTEIN (1945) emphasize that Asclepius carried out surgical procedures which contemporary physicians would not have attempted. And he applied medicines that others were unable to apply. The evidence presented by EDELSTEIN/EDELSTEIN (1945) refers to reports from Epidaurus which are undoubtedly of a miraculous nature. The fact that they were edited by the priests in itself renders these reports dubious. The prescriptions, on the other hand, include information on baths, exercise and medicines (above all herbal medicines) which are all closely related to the contemporary medical thinking as reflected in the specialist literature (KRUG 1993: 141). The Emperor Marcus Aurelius himself provided evidence of these prescriptions because he adhered to the therapies he heard about in his dream, as did his teacher Fronto and his friend, Aelius Aristides (M. AUR. 5.8 and ARTEM. 4.22). Another instructive example is the Epidaurian votive inscription by M. Iulius Apellas (second century CE), a member of a prominent family in Mylasa, a city in the region of Caria in Asia Minor (IG IV² 1.126 and Steger 2000: 30 with note 12). The instruction this patient received in his dream attests to a medical procedure that was similar to those commonly used at the time (III.5.2). EDELSTEIN/EDELSTEIN (1945) already called attention to the parallels they discovered with the contemporary medicine. KRUG's peculiar deliberations on psychosomatics in this context (1993: 140 f.) should be dropped and more attention be given to the rational-scientific aspects described in Apellas' account of his therapies. KRUG's restrictive statements cannot prove either that the Epidaurian healing reports were mostly subjective accounts. The conclusions regarding the healing cult or medicine therefore also need to be called into question. The cult personnel assisted in implementing the instructions received by the patients, whether they referred to baths, physical exercise or sacrifices, but also beyond that.

In summary we can say that two types of dreams need to be distinguished in evaluating the sources available. One type refers to the kind of faith healings that are also known from Christian accounts of miraculous cures and that were used for propagandistic purposes to support the image of "the emperor as healer". Secondly there are the reports resulting from the dreams which were written down as a token of gratitude toward Asclepius. They preserve the medical instructions given in the practice of Asclepius. Representative examples of the latter type can serve to support the thesis presented above regarding a separate Asclepian medicine.

III.4 – Methodological considerations

The reports of cures given by patients are specific to particular cultures and social structures, as we have shown in chapter III.2 which dealt with the social construction of illness (LACHMUND/STOLLBERG 1992). The afflictions described and the measures recommended in the medical reports cannot be described in modern terms, nor can they be diagnosed or interpreted retrospectively. What we can do is analyze the disease process from the point of view of medical history (LEVEN 1998/2004). Condoning retrospective diagnosis in the history of medicine would be equivalent to accepting anachronistic methods in history. For a meaningful, representative and medical-historical analysis aspects such as the respective contemporary views of illness and of the origin of an illness, need to be taken into account. This approach was most recently opposed by GRAUMANN (2000) who, based on a synopsis of the case histories in the Hippocratic Books on Epidemics, called LEVEN's methodical criticism of GRMEK (1989) into question. He collated the (retrospective) diagnoses established by scholars between 1875 and 1998 (760 individual diagnoses by 80 authors) for this purpose. However, his "mediating" proposal regarding retrospective diagnosis is not convincing. Moreover, the case histories in question provide information not only on diseases but on other aspects, too, and they are often valuable sources of knowledge when it comes to details of everyday culture. The Books on Epidemics do not give us any insight into the inner state of the patients and can therefore not be used for analysis in the history of patients (STEGER 2007).

As early as 1985, the British social historian ROY PORTER demanded in a programmatic essay entitled "The patient's view: doing medical history from below" that illness, healers, and their environment should no longer be examined from the physicians' perspective but increasingly from that of the patients. PORTER's postulate constitutes a methodological turning point in medical history and shows that the subjective turnaround in history is also noticeable in medical sociology (JÜTTE 1990). By now the methodological approach of patient history has in itself become the subject of scientific inquiry. WOLFF (1998a/1998b) has compiled the varying perspectives of patient historiography. The history of patients as a cultural-historical turning point in medical historiography has been investigated by ERNST (1998). In patient research we have to differentiate between the role of the patient on the one hand and the assessment of socio-structural data of patients on the other. The socio-scientific approach is particularly problematic when it comes to ancient medicine. WOLFF (1998a: 316–319) stresses that this is a patient-oriented research question which contributes to the socio-medical history by means of quantifying and statistical procedures. PORTER (1985a) initially referred to the history of patients as "terra incognita." Two programmatic volumes followed (PORTER/PORTER 1988 and PORTER 1985b). We can now say that the history of patients is no longer unknown territory (STEGER 2007 and DINGES 2002b). Most recently, ISRAELOWICH (2015) devoted himself to the patient-physician relationship in the Roman imperial period.

PORTER's appeal can best be followed by studying the thank-offerings donated to the Asclepieia by patients, because these testimonies reveal their view of the procedures applied there. This approach focuses less on the medical thinking (GRMEK 1996) to which the investigation into ancient medical history has so far been limited but rather on the patient as a thinking and acting subject. In the context of cultural history, and based on CLIFFORD GEERTZ' idea of a "thick description," medicine can be seen as a "network of relationships that is defined and shaped at a particular time and that includes various groups of agents," with "patients only ever [constituting] a part of a close-ly-knit web of agents involved in the healthcare processes" (WOLFF 1998a: 312 and 315). The concept of "medical culture", which is often cited in this context, should be called to mind (ROELCKE 1998). A history of patients needs to ask about the implementation, diffusion and reception of medical ideas. It is no longer the person performing the act of healing who is of primary interest but the recipients of these actions: the analysis of their perception complements the existing knowledge. On the basis of the behavioural patterns that are now at the centre of the inquiry the attempt can be made to find access to the pa-tients' inner experiences (WOLFF 1998a: 324). But: however innovative and fruitful the methodical approach of the history of patients may be, using the term "patient" is problematic because it presupposes professionality (WOLFF 1998a: 313 f.).

The type of text best suited to the research into illness from the patient's point of view is autobiographical and self-reflective (autobiographies, mem-oirs, diaries). Self-reflective documents yield rich insights into the diverse as-pects of dealing with illness, the subjective experience of illness, the ways in which help was sought, and particularly also the confrontation with "alterna-tive" approaches. The individual experience of illness and the patient's mental and emotional reflection on his or her sick body are both subject to historical change. On the one hand, the experiences of illness are tinted by individual perception and can therefore contribute to the history of the body, particu-larly when it comes to the experience of pain (KING 2017). On the other hand, these experiences are subject to numerous socio-cultural factors and therefore instructive documents on everyday culture. Descriptions of the experience of illness are informed by social circumstances. Experiences of illness are influ-enced by collective social patterns as well as by the individual patients' body memories. WOLFF divides the questions relevant to the history of patients into various categories: patient health and social circumstances, the relationship between patients and other health-related agents, the behaviours of patients regarding illness and health, or the regaining of health, and the patients' ideas on questions of health (WOLFF 1998a: 319–323).

So far research has been mostly restricted to the sources reaching back to the early modern period, while the time prior to that has hardly been con-sidered. Noteworthy in this respect is the research carried out at the Institute for the History of Medicine of the Robert Bosch Foundation in Stuttgart (Germany). JÜTTE (1991) used this approach in a fruitful way in his work on everyday medicine in the early modern period. LACHMUND/STOLLBERG

(1995) presented a basic study derived from autobiographies from the eighteenth century and later. JANKRIFT (2003) has studied earlier periods, investigating, for instance, the situation of lepers as reflected in late-medieval and early modern leprosy confirmation reports and personal testimonials. I already outlined the limits and opportunities of a patient-focused history of ancient medicine (STEGER 2007). Recently, a collection was published by PETRIDOU/THUMIGER (2016) on the history of patients in antiquity. It has been stated, quite rightly, that studying the history of patients is particularly demanding because the sources are difficult to access and interpret and the investigative methods are limited (WOLFF 1998a: 311). A (historically unique) example of analysis based on the methods of patient history is the practice of Samuel Hahnemann (1755–1843) (DINGES 2002a). The history of homeopathy is particularly suited to be examined from the point of view of the history of patients because of the patient journals and the large number of patient letters which yield much more information on their social milieus (JÜTTE 1996).

For Antiquity in particular, the required focus on the patients can only be honoured to a limited extent, mainly because, in most cases, no documents survive that could count as patient information. As has been pointed out before, the extensive material of the Hippocratic Corpus is not really suited to answer the questions arising in the history of patients: although the books on epidemics contain – aside from climatic descriptions and aphorisms – also case histories, these original testimonials were not composed by the patients but by the physicians who treated them. In addition, the votive offerings and donations are not necessarily of a self-reflective nature and most of them are rather concise which means that the information that can be gleaned from them is limited, as the following examples will show. Publius Aelius Aristides, a prominent patient at the Asclepieion in Pergamum, who will be discussed in more detail below, sent servants with an inscription to the sanctuary at Pergamum. In this case, Aristides made a donation because he wanted to make sure that his speech would go well. This donation would be a suitable source for patient-oriented questions but it has unfortunately not been preserved. The inscription of Diogenes, a Lycian from Oinoanda (120 CE), on the other hand, is a self-reflective document that even contains a protreptic in favour of therapeutic reflection based on self-experience (STEGER 2004: 187 f. and SMITH 2003/2000/1996/1993). However, this kind of inscription is unique. A search of the sources available reveals that there are only few objects that yield substantial information. It also needs to be considered that votive gifts constitute a separate group which is distinct from others primarily because of political influences and economic circumstances. What we do not have are extensive bodies of sources reflecting the patients' perspective. There are nonetheless some individual testimonies which are relatively instructive. Micro-historical case studies could be the method of choice. Micro-observation does not focus on general or historical details but on the way they are imbedded in their wider context. This kind of inquiry into individual actions, experiences and real life situations can yield insights into socio-cultural networks and the way they relate to each other. The much-cited contrast between the micro-historical and the macro-historical approaches (SCHLUMBOHM 1998) needs to be reconsidered and both approaches be integrated in the examination "of individuals and the ways they interact with and depend on each other." (MEDICK 2001: 88)

Patient introspections can also be found in the literary sources, as the following analysis of Aristides' *Hieroi Logoi* will demonstrate (STEGER 2012). The problems we meet here are connected with questions of fictiveness and subjective colouring, both of which can be overcome with a critical approach on the one hand and thorough scrutiny of perceptions, interpretations and underlying ideas on the other.

III.5 – The patients of Asclepius

III.5.1 – P. Aelius Aristides at Pergamum

As has been pointed out earlier, self-reflective documents were produced in the context of the practice of Asclepius, the God of healing, and these documents can provide valuable information on Asclepian medicine from the patients' point of view. A large body of material was left by Publius Aelius Aristides, the Greek sophist and orator, who spent several years at Pergamum as a patient of Asclepius.

Aristides was born at Hadriani in Mysia, a region in Asia Minor (MUDRY 1989, PEARCY 1988, SCHRÖDER 1986: 9 f. and KLEIN 1983: 71). Thanks to the details provided in his horoscope (ARISTEID. hier. log. 4.58) the birth of Aristides can be dated precisely to 26 November 117 CE (BEHR 1969). He was born into a wealthy family of which he says little, however. When his father Eudaimon, a priest of Zeus, died Aristides inherited a considerable fortune that gave him social security and financial independence. The extensive educational journeys he undertook, to Egypt for instance (FRON 2014), provide ample information on his social circumstances.

Out of gratitude to Asclepius, Aristides, "an invalid orator struggling to discover the meaning of his life" (SCHRÖDER 1988), left behind a detailed patient journal which, in his own words, was named "ἱεροὶ λόγοι" by Asclepius himself (2.9):

(…) διαλεχθείη [sc. ὁ θεός] (…) ἄλλα τε δή, οἶμαι, καὶ ὅτι ἐπισημήναιτο ὡδὶ λέγων· ἱεροὶ λόγοι.
(…) among other comments the God, I think, also gave them his blessings by calling them "Sacred Tales".

Aristides began writing these discourses on his Laneion estate (BEHR 1968: 116–130) in the winter of 170/171 CE, some time after his therapeutic sojourn at Pergamum and based on the notes he had made there. Right at the beginning, he said, the god had instructed him to record his dreams (2.2) and now he was able to make recourse to the notes which he had written himself or dictated when he was unable to write.

Aristides' writings offer in-depth information on the healthcare provided at Pergamum. Historians need to approach them with care because they comprise, for the most part, the biased and embellished eulogies of a hypochondriac worshipper of Asclepius. Nevertheless, the *hieroi logoi* are more than just reflections of Aristides' pious adoration of Asclepius, because they supply the careful investigator with valuable information on the healthcare provided at Pergamum during the imperial period. Aside from the *hieroi logoi*, which consist of six sacred tales, Aristides also left orations on Asclepius, the springs and the water of Pergamum (RUSSELL/TRAPP/NESSELRATH 2016). The medical historian who studies his prose hymns more closely (or. 38; 39; 42 and 53) will find this a sobering experience, however. As inside sources for a medical historian's investigation into everyday Asclepian medicine they are of limited value; but they open up rich insights into the religious rituals in an Asclepian sanctuary (STEGER 2016b). The hymn *The Sons of Asclepius*, for instance, speaks of the family of Asclepius (38.6 ff.) and the diffusion of the Asclepian cult (38.21). Interestingly, the hymn begins with a citation from the Iliad that mentions a dream as the source of this tale, evoking the dreams which are so crucial to the cult and medicine of Asclepius and which are proof of the contact between the devotee, or patient, and Asclepius in a "rite of passage". The oration *"On the Fountain in the Temple of Asclepius"* is an homage to sacred sites. It describes how the fountain, like a drug, gives the supplicants what they need (39.14). Unfortunately it does not say anything essential about the medicine as such. It highlights the special significance of water (39.12 ff.), which is in fact central to the Asclepian cult and medicine (39.15 f. and STEGER 2005b). The strength of Aristides' bond with Asclepius is apparent at the very beginning of the *Hymn to Asclepius* which, in style, is strongly reminiscent of the *hieroi logoi* (42.1). Further investigation of this hymn fails to yield more detailed information on the patient's inner experience. Nevertheless, this hymn is the source from which the history of medicine can glean most insights: on the Asclepieia, where therapies were administered day and night (42.5), on the dietetic instructions which were part of the therapy and closely related to the contemporary medical ideas, on the effects they may have had on others (42.8), and also on Aristides' personal experience with these instructions (42.10). Finally, in *Eulogy on the Waters of Pergamum*, a hymn of which only fragments have been preserved, Aristides speaks of a dream that revealed the significance of the Pergamene water, which is central to the Asclepian cult and medicine (53.3). The value of these hymns as sources can be compared – by anyone wishing to attempt such a comparison – with Lucian of Samosata's *Alexander or the False Prophet*. Lucian's *Alexander* can be used fruitfully to enhance the understanding of the imperial history of religion – it is a key source for the cult of Asclepius at Abonuteichus – but when it comes to the actual medical practice it yields only a few rudimentary statements. While the historical analysis of *Alexander* can cast light on the healing cult at Abonuteichus and the connection between religion and medicine, it does not provide a clearer picture of the nature of Asclepian medicine (STEGER 2005a). Similarly with Aristides' prose hymns: the medical historian cannot glean much information from them on the history of Asclepian medicine.

BEHR (1968) has presented a monograph based on good factual knowledge and careful inquiry. His work is today considered the standard reference on the life and work of Aristides. In addition to the writings on Aristides' complete works within their contemporary context (BITTRICH 2016 and SWAIN 1996: 254–297) ISRAELOWICH (2012) has submitted the most recent in-depth investigation of the *hieroi logoi*. His study focuses mainly on their value as sources of medical history and on their integration into the imperial healthcare system. Here, Aristides appears as an informed patient, a view that is in opposition to KORENJAK (2005), who proposes that Aristides' accounts of therapies go against any medical τέχνη. He argues that Aristides, as a representative of the "Second Sophistic" (RICHTER/JOHNSON 2017), the contemporary school of oratory, tried to distinguish himself with his writings. Whether the divine instructions are indeed opposed to the imperial medicine is doubtful, as we will see later. PETSALIS-DIOMIDIS (2010) rehabilitates Aristides by showing that this seemingly bizarre private text is in fact an eloquent expression of religious experience, and by placing him in the medical-cultic context of the Pergamene Asclepieion. However, she does not consider STEGER's findings (2004).

The *Hieroi Logoi*, to which Philostratus (soph. 581), in his *Lives of the Sophists*, referred as "sacred books," belong to the most comprehensive introspective accounts we have because they record Aristides' experience of his own body on an almost daily basis (1.3):

ἑκάστη γὰρ τῶν ἡμετέρων ἡμερῶν, ὡσαύτως δὲ καὶ νυκτῶν, ἔχει συγγραφήν, εἴ τις παρ᾽
ἓν ἢ τὰ συμπίπτοντα ἀπογράφειν ἠβούλετο ἢ τὴν τοῦ θεοῦ πρόνοιαν διηγεῖσθαι, ὧν τὰ
μὲν ἐκ τοῦ φανεροῦ παρών, τὰ δὲ τῇ πομπῇ· τῶν ἐνυπνίων, ἐνεδείκνυτο, ὅσα γε δὴ καὶ
ὕπνου λαχεῖν ἐξῆν· σπάνιον δ᾽ ἦν ὑπὸ τῶν περὶ τὸ σῶμα τρικυμιῶν.

For each of my days as well as each of my nights has its own history, if only someone
who was there could write down the occurrences or describe the care that the god
displayed partly by appearing personally or by sending dream images, to the extent
that it was given to me to find sleep. But this happened rarely in the surges of my
physical constitutions.

At the very beginning of Book I Aristides provides an in-depth account over a period of six weeks (1.4–57) of his physical condition and of how he experienced his therapies and his body. His oration on the God of Healing offers comprehensive material which contains, in addition to his introspections, what he himself (1.16) calls "appendage" (παρέργον). The therapies he had at Pergamum between 143 and 157 CE are part of this. Speaking of the baths prescribed to him by the god in Pergamum (2.71–80), he described, for instance, also his incubation experience. The significance of incubations has been discussed in the chapter on the architecture of the sanctuaries (III.2). Aristides anointed himself in an open courtyard within the sanctuary walls and bathed in the holy fountain. According to the reconstruction of the incubation process, the worshippers washed first so they would be pure when entered the temple precinct. Archaeological excavations at Pergamum confirmed that there was a holy spring in front of the temple precinct. From there the bathing houses, which were fed by the spring water, were already visible (KRUG 1993: 167). The cleansing before entering the sacred precinct was an essential aspect of the incubation ritual and was followed by sacrifices and prayers, before the patients would lie down to sleep inside the temple. Aristides relates how he, as instructed in a dream, lay down between the portal and the lattice gates of the temple (2.71).

These first intimations seem to indicate that Aristides' ego-documents provide an ideal "inside view" of his body-experience as well as a view "from below" into the healthcare provided at Pergamum – certainly at first glance. If we study his descriptions more closely, however, we notice that they are often exaggerated, distorted, even fictitious.

Take, as a first example, Aristides' dream (1.23), in which he relates how, coming from Phrygia, he and his teacher, Alexander of Cotiaeum, met Antoninus Pius and his entourage: the emperor was astonished that Aristides did not greet him in the customary way with a friendly kiss. Aristides explained his omission by pointing out that he worshipped Asclepius who had instructed him not to cultivate other friendships (1.23). Antoninus Pius accepted this explanation, agreeing that the adoration of Asclepius surpassed any other. This episode, which is usually ascribed to Aristides' first sojourn in Rome in 144 CE, is probably pure fiction – a thesis that is corroborated on the one hand by the highly embellished form in which he presents the dream, and also by the fact that – according to parallel accounts – Aristides did not yet have such an intimate relationship with Asclepius in 144 CE. It is moreover very unlikely that he would have had the audacity to speak to the emperor in this way and to give priority to Asclepius (SCHRÖDER 1986: 26 note 46). PERNOT (2008: 178 f.) thought the episode was a deliberate illustration of the aloofness of the Greek Aristides towards the Romans. Potential fictionality plays no part in this interpretation. Another argument in favour of Aristides having exaggerated and distorted the truth is his claim that he pleaded with Asclepius to help him with composing his orations (2.4). He asked Asclepius (2.24) in which order he should present the events so they would please the God and promote his own progress. Whether there is any truth to Aristides' notes considering his need for muse-like inspiration, which is reminiscent rather of epic or lyrical traditions, needs to be critically investigated. Homer, in his *Iliad* and *Odyssey*, also appealed to the muse for inspiration. Aristides' tendency to exaggerate is also apparent when he writes how working on his manuscript caused him the greatest agony (4.22), that he was unable to breathe and struggled to regain consciousness.

The detailed precision of his descriptions, of the dreams in particular, which has provoked such doubts as to the reliability of his statements, was certainly to an extent also due to the great expectations of the supplicants (SCHRÖDER 1986: 13 and BEHR 1968: 116) which focused on the incubations and the healing people hoped they would bring. Aristides, the worshipper and patient, placed all his hopes in Asclepius seeing that the physicians in Rome and in Smyrna had been unable to help him (2.7):

ἐνταῦθα πρῶτον ὁ Σωτὴρ χρηματίζειν ἤρξατο· ἀνυπόδητόν τε γὰρ προελθεῖν ἐπέταξεν καὶ ἐβόων δὴ ἐν τῷ ὀνείρατι ὡς ἂν ὕπαρ τε καὶ ἐπ᾽ ὀνείρατι τετελεσμένῳ ‘μέγας ὁ Ἀσκληπιός· τετέλεσται τὸ πρόσταγμα᾽.

Now the healer ("soter") began his revelations for the first time. And he ordered me to walk barefoot. And so I cried out in my dream, as if I were awake, and after the dream was fulfilled, "Great is Asclepius! His will has been done."

Aristides' devotion to Asclepius is also apparent from the description of his miraculous salvation from dangers (2.24–36) which he owed, as he explains, to the interference of the deity (2.25).

This precision, which is often judged to be exaggerated, is not only a result of the strong focus placed by the devotees on the procedure itself, but also of the wide-spread knowledge of remedies and diets. This also explains the well-documented and precise ideas in relation to questions of health: Aristides mentions particular salves, medicines and dietary instructions (3.21–37 and BEHR 1968: 162–170). One of the medicines prescribed for him by Asclepius was a balm to which he refers as the gift of Telesphorus (2.10). Another was the royal ointment (3.21) that had a soothing effect on throat problems and tensions radiating out from the ear. Asclepius recommended to Aristides that he should use this ointment, and that he should receive it from a woman. He was given the medicine in the sanctuary at the feet of Hygieia, where Tyche had deposited it. He applied this ointment and was relieved of his spasms soon afterwards (3.22). He casually reveals more information about the composition of the salves (3.23):

(…) ὅτι εἴη κρᾶσις τριῶν, ὁποῦ τε ᾧ χριόμεθα καὶ μύρου ναρδίνου καὶ ἑτέρου μύρου τῶν πολυτελῶν, ἔστιν δ᾽, οἶμαι, τοῦ φύλλου ἐπώνυμον.
(…) it was a mixture of three components: the juice [of the balm tree], with which we anoint ourselves, of nard oil and another precious oil which, I believe, is named after the leaf [from which it is extracted].

More detailed information about the composition that was used in a soaking compress is given by GALEN (De simpl. medicament. temp. 13.184 K.). The φάρμακον βασιλικόν (τετραφάρμακον) and its four ingredients (cera, resina, pix and adeps) are also mentioned elsewhere (GAL. De elem. sec. Hipp. 1.452 K; De simpl. medicament. temp. 12.328 K., and SCHRÖDER 1986: 69 note 34). In this context Aristides gives numerous individual examples from his own experience with the deity and he states that Asclepius not only prescribed remedies he prepared himself but also those that could be bought on the market

(3.30). From this description the reader learns something about the forms of therapy recommended by Asclepius, which apparently included surgical interventions as well as pharmaceutical therapies (4.64):

> (...) ταύτῃ μοι ἐδόκει ὁ ἱερεὺς, ὁ τοῦ Ἀσκληπιοῦ οὗτος, ὁ ἔτι νῦν ὤν, καὶ ὁ τούτου πάππος, ἐφ᾽ οὗ τὰ πολλὰ καὶ μεγάλα, ὡς ἐπυνθανόμεθα, ἐχειρούργησεν ὁ θεός (...).
>
> (...) the priest of Asclepius then appeared to me, the one in office now and his grandfather, during whose tenure, as we find out, the god conducted numerous major operations (...)

The grandfather of the priest Asclepiacos was Flavius Asclepiades, who was a priest to Asclepius at Pergamum in the first century CE. If Aristides is to be believed, surgical interventions were carried out in Pergamum at that time. Even if one can explain the scrupulous descriptions with a particular focus on the procedure as such and with an extensive medical knowledge, it is still possible that the tales are fictitious. There is for instance the implausible request made of Aristides by Asclepius, namely that he should have 120 *litroi* of blood drawn from his body – a quantity that corresponds to about 33 litres. This is an obvious exaggeration seeing that an adult male has only 4.5 to 6 litres of blood in his system (SCHRÖDER 1986: 54 note 89). Aristides himself often speaks of miraculous tales when he mentions events that are related to Asclepius (2.74): in the winter of 144 CE, for instance, he was only able to take a bath in Smyrna because the rain stopped for a short period of time, a miraculous feat, he thought, that only Asclepius could have achieved (2.50). A similar marvel occurred when he was about to take a bath at Pergamum and Asclepius – miraculously – provided enough water for even three baths (2.51–53). And again, it was only possible for Aristides to take a bath in Elaea, the port of Pergamum, because Asclepius worked a miracle (2.54–56).

At first glance Aristides' account seems to be a veritable treasure, offering an inner perspective of the social milieu and the healthcare provided at Pergamum supported by countless details. The reservations mentioned show, however, that Aristides – particularly because he had such an intimate relationship with Asclepius – provides a picture of the events at the sanctuary that is, at least in parts, misleading and not free from fiction. Scholars intent on evaluating Aristides' narratives for a history of the medical provisions at Pergamum need to be aware of this particular circumstance. Leaving these problematic sources entirely out of the picture, on the other hand, would mean ignoring valuable reflections of a famous patient of Asclepius. A history of patients can find in these tales glimpses of a patient's inner experiences, his dealings with healers, physicians, and – in this case – with Asclepius, the God of Healing, furthermore of the resulting controversies and conflicts, the mutual appreciation and repudiation, and plenty of other socio-historical details. Considering this wealth of information further analysis of Aristides' Tales is certainly worthwhile:

In the winter of 144 CE Aristides travelled to Rome where he hoped to be introduced to the imperial family. The journey to Rome proved extremely difficult, because he suffered from fever and respiratory problems. In retrospect he wrote that, on his way to Rome, he contracted many illnesses, of which his choking fits were the most dangerous (2.5 f.):

ἐπειδὴ γὰρ ἐκομίσθην ἀπὸ τῆς Ἰταλίας, πολλὰ καὶ παντοῖα συνειλοχὼς τῷ σώματι ἀπὸ τῶν συνεχῶν καμάτων τε καὶ χειμώνων, οἷς ἐχρησάμην ἀπιὼν διὰ Θρᾴκης καὶ Μακεδονίας, ἔτι κάμνων ἐξελθὼν οἴκοθεν (…) χαλεπώτατον δ᾽ ἁπάντων καὶ ἀπορώτατον ὅτι τοῦ πνεύματος ἀπεκεκλείμην καὶ μετὰ πολλῆς τῆς πραγματείας καὶ ἀπιστίας μόλις ἄν ποτε ἀνέπνευσα βιαίως καὶ ἀγαπητῶς, πνιγμοί τε παρηκολούθουν συνεχεῖς ἐν τῷ τραχήλῳ καὶ τὰ νεῦρα ἐπεφρίκει καὶ σκέπης ἔδει πλείονος ἢ φέρειν δυνατὸς ἦν· χωρὶς δ᾽ ἕτερα ἀμύθητα ἠνώχλει.

When I was taken home from Italy (by ship), I had contracted various physical afflictions due to the permanent strains and storms I had to face on my way (to Rome) via Thrace and Macedonia. I was ill even as I left home (…) The most ill-fated and hazardous of them all were the choking fits, during which I rarely and only with the greatest effort and hopelessness managed to force a breath, and (the fact) that I had permanent cramps of the throat, that I suffered chills and shivers and needed more covers than I could bear. In addition, I had other immense pains.

Later, when he was at Allianoi, Aristides was still complaining, doubting that he would live to see the day when he was released from his great suffering. Recently, KING (2017: 129–155) devoted a whole chapter to Aristides in his history of pain in Greek culture under the Roman Empire. It turned out that Aristides' descriptions of experiencing pain and illness fit very well with other representations of medical experience of his era. PHILOSTRATUS, his biographer, tells us that Aristides was generally of a sickly constitution (soph. 2.9), but his anecdotal tales also need to be read with caution (SWAIN 1991).

As we can gather from Aristides' descriptions, the dreams and dream reports were central to the therapeutic program at Pergamum (2.8). Aristides mentions more than a hundred dreams that brought healing to his body and soul (2.8):

εἰ δέ τις τὰ ἀκριβέστατα γνῶναι βουλήσεται τῶν γεγενημένων ἡμῖν παρὰ τοῦ θεοῦ, ὥρα τὰς διφθέρας αὐτῷ ζητεῖν καὶ τὰ ὀνείρατα αὐτά. καὶ γὰρ ἰάματα παντὸς εἴδους καὶ διαλόγους τινὰς εὑρήσει καὶ λόγους ἐν μήκει καὶ φάσματα αντοῖα καὶ προρρήσεις ἁπάσας καὶ χρησμῳ-δίας περὶ παντοδαπῶν πραγμάτων, τὰς μὲν καταλογάδην, τὰς δὲ ἐν μέτροις γεγονυίας, καὶ χαρίτων πάντ᾽ ἄξια τῷ θεῷ μειζόνων ἤ τις ἂν εἰκάσαι.

Anyone wishing to know the exact circumstances of the deeds the God performed on me needs to consult the parchments and the dream reports themselves. There, he will find remedies of all kinds, some conversations and detailed speeches, phenomena and prophecies and oracles of all kinds about the most diverse questions, some in prose, others in verse, all demanding the utmost gratitude towards the God.

The dreams provide more information about the therapy at the Asclepieion. Aside from remedies, conversations and speeches, they also contain oracles and prophecies. We know that the physicians had the greatest respect for these dreams. Once, Aristides was apparently approached by a physician (1.57) who wanted to help him but changed his mind when Aristides told him about his dream. The physician explained his behaviour by pointing out that he had sense enough to make way for the God. From this Aristides drew the conclusion that none but Asclepius could be "his" physician. Asclepius alone was able to free him from his afflictions. In another situation, the physician Theodotus prescribed a therapy for Aristides based on the dream images sent by Asclepius (4.38). This physician advised Aristides to have boys sing some of his songs to him and he was indeed freed from his pain.

Aristides describes a great number of symptoms and illnesses that tormented him on his journeys (2.60–62 and BEHR 1968: 165–168). When he travelled to Rome in the middle of winter – having been sick even as he set off – he suffered the most terrible earache and was generally in a poor state of health, which was further aggravated by coughs and excessive stress (2.62):

καὶ τοῦτο μὲν περὶ τῶν ὀδόντων ἐν παντὶ κατέστην, ὥσθ᾽ ὑπεῖχον τὰς χεῖρας, ὡς αἰεὶ δεξόμε-νος, τροφῆς δὲ καὶ παντάπασιν ἀπεκεκλείμην, ὅτι μὴ γάλακτος μόνου· τοῦ τε ἄσθματος περὶ τὸ στῆθος ᾐσθόμην τότε πρῶτον καὶ πυρετοὶ κατέλαβον ἰσχυροὶ καὶ ἄλλα ἀμύθητα·
First my teeth gave me the utmost discomfort so that I held my hand in front of my mouth ready to catch them. I was unable to take in anything but milk. It was the first time that I experienced the breathlessness in my chest, and I was plagued with severe fever and indescribable other afflictions.

It needed the greatest effort to reach Rome at all after a hundred days of travelling. Once he was there, he complained that all his inner organs were swollen, that his nerves were rigid with cold and that he had great difficulty breathing. Once he was in Rome Aristides was unable to recover fully although he underwent, as he said, extended and painful treatment (2.63 f.). The doctors gave him sharp purgatives which resulted in a bloody diarrhoea. In addition he developed such a high fever that he gave up all hope of improvement. The doctors made incisions all over his body from his chest to his bladder and even cupped him. He became extremely breathless and suffered agonies of pain. No one was able to help him (2.63):

καὶ πάντα αἵματι ἐπέφυρτο καὶ γίγνομαι ὑπέρινος, καὶ τῶν σπλάγχων ᾐσθανόμην οἷον ψυχρῶν τε καὶ ἐκκρεμαμένων, καὶ τὸ τῆς ἀμηχανίας τῆς περὶ τὴν ἀναπνοὴν ἐπετάθη.
Everything was smeared with blood and I was purged excessively. I felt that my bowels were cold and that they were hanging down (lifelessly), and my breathlessness worsened.

These few examples prove once more how well-suited Aristides' descriptions are to the study of the history of patients in general: they provide insights into Aristides' behaviour with regard to illness and health, or the regaining of health, and into his relationship with other health-related agents. For instance, he speaks in rather a deprecatory manner about the physicians in Rome and also in Smyrna (2.5 and BEHR 1968: 162–170): in Smyrna not only the physicians were unable to help him; bathing in the hot springs and his prayers to Serapis were also in vain. Aristides then decided to seek out Asclepius at Pergamum and there – this much can be anticipated – he found a therapy that helped him. The dream reports suggest that Aristides had a very intimate relationship with Asclepius: Asclepius was "his" God (4.50) and "his" physician (1.57). From then on Aristides placed his trust only in physicians who yielded whole-heartedly to the "true physician."

The very first cures prescribed by Asclepius (2.11–23) brought improvement: at Smyrna Asclepius instructed Aristides to take a bath in the river that flowed past the city (2.18). He did as he was told and bathed in the pleasantly warm water of the river (2.21). As he climbed out of the water he felt a great lightness of body and he thanked Asclepius. This sense of wellbeing lingered until bedtime and the warmth pervaded his entire body. He also experienced an incredible mental serenity and harmony. By following the advice of Asclepius to take a bath at Smyrna, Aristides therefore improved in body and soul. We also find out that Aristides was so grateful to Asclepius that he ac-

cepted the name "Theodorus" from him (PETSALIS-DIOMIDIS 2010: 132–150).
Asclepius had – to a certain extent and for a certain period of time – healed
him from his long-standing ailments (4.53; 4.70) and Aristides felt, as the
name Theodorus suggests, that he had received a gift from god (4.53):

καὶ μὴν τοὔνομά γε ὁ Θεόδωρος οὕτως ἐπωνομάσθη μοι. προσρηθῆναι μὲν ἔδοξα ὡς
ἐν Σμύρνῃ ὑπό τινος καὶ μάλα συγχαίροντος· 'Θεόδωρε χαῖρε' – καὶ Ἀσιάρχης', οἶμαι,
προσῆν –, δέξασθαι δὲ οὕτω τὴν πρόσρησιν, ὡς ἄρα πᾶν τοὐμὸν εἴη τοῦ θεοῦ δωρέα.

I was also given the name of Theodorus in the following way. It seemed as if someone
addressed me at Smyrna with warm blessings, saying, "Greetings, Theodorus!" – I
think he added the epithet "Asiarches" as well – and I understood the address to
signify that all I am and own is a gift of god.

We find out in this context that Aristides had refrained from bathing for more
than five years (1.59) and that he only bathed in the sea, in a river or spring
after receiving the corresponding instructions from Asclepius, mostly in the
winter. In addition he had, during the previous two years and two months,
endured the purging of his upper respiratory tract with enemas and blood-let-
ting. He was particularly upset about the extent of this treatment and the poor
food inflicted on him during that time. Despite his severe criticism Aristides
did not question the therapies imposed on him while he was in such a desperate situation. Rather than with enlightened reflection he responded with the
willing acceptance of divine instructions.

The concrete dilemmas resulting from this situation are described by
Aristides in the discourse on "Hernia and Dropsy" (1.61–68): he suffered from
a swelling that kept growing and caused him great distress (1.63). His friends
knew about this and some admired his steadfastness. Others, when they saw
him suffer, reprimanded him for relying too much on his dreams. Others again
accused him of being afraid of medicines and of the knife. Aristides' illness
was so far advanced that he even had to make his speeches from his sickbed.
Asclepius, he said, had repeatedly demanded of him that he should practise
his oratory skills. While he was at Pergamum he started practising again even
though he found this very difficult (4.22), but he soon experienced real therapeutic successes (4.15–19). While Aristides complained about weakness, discomfort and breathing difficulties at the beginning of his oratory practice, he
improved in the course of his training. Declaiming strengthened his health
and gave him new energy (4.24). Making speeches even helped against his
toothache (4.30). Because Aristides' situation was so desperate, and because
his tumour kept growing, Asclepius now appeared and recommended a ther-

apy (1.66). Soon the patient improved and the physicians could only marvel at the wonderful care provided by the God (1.66).

τέλος δὲ ὁ Σωτὴρ σημαίνει τῆς αὐτῆς νυκτὸς ταὐτὸν ἐμοί τε καὶ τῷ τροφεῖ – περιῆν γὰρ δὴ τότε ὁ Ζώσιμος –, ὥστε ἐγὼ μὲν ἔπεμπον ἐκείνῳ φράσων ἅ εἰρηκὼς εἴη ὁ θεός, ὁ δ᾽ ἀπήντα φράσων αὐτός μοι ἅ ἠκηκόει τοῦ θεοῦ· ἦν δέ τι φάρμακον οὗ τὰ μὲν καθ᾽ ἕκαστα οὐ μέμνημαι, ἀλλὰ δὲ ὅτι μετεῖχεν· ὡς δὲ ἐπεπάσαμεν, ἔρρει δὴ ταχὺ τοῦ ὄγκου τὸ πλεῖστον, καὶ ἅμα ἕῳ παρῆσαν οἱ ἐπιτήδειοι χαίροντες μετὰ ἀπιστίας.

In the end the healer ("soter") made the same revelation to me and my foster-father (Zosimus was then still alive) in the same night, so that I sent forth a messenger informing him what the God had said, while he himself met the messenger and asked him to tell me what he had heard from the God. It was a remedy, however, of which I do not recall the individual parts. I only remember that salt was one of them. When we had applied it the swelling soon disappeared and at the break of day, my friends were there, joyful and incredulous at the same time.

The physicians then discussed the wonderful cure granted by Asclepius and how the hole left by the tumour could be filled. They recommended that Aristides should undergo surgery because the wound would not heal otherwise. Asclepius, however, contradicted the physicians and recommended to apply an egg to the wound. Again Asclepius proved to be right and again the physicians had to give in to his superior knowledge. We learn here not only what kinds of therapy were available to Aristides but also how diverse they were.

Aristides had to deal with the views of the physicians which mostly contradicted the instructions of Asclepius, the true physician and god of healing. The demands of Asclepius, moreover, often caused tensions as is apparent from Aristides' account of how he was advised against eating beef in Smyrna in the spring of 149 CE (3.37): an oracle had appeared to his servant Zosimus telling him that he would live as long as the cow was grazing in the field. The oracle also advised Zosimus to stay away from beef altogether. Zosimus was apparently not consistent enough because he is said to have died from eating beef (1.69–77; 3.47–50). This caused a dilemma for Aristides when he was expected to sacrifice a cow (3.39): When a devastating earthquake destroyed Mytilene on the island of Lesbos and caused severe damage in Smyrna and Ephesus, Asclepius demanded the sacrifice of a cow from Aristides. Thinking of the oracle and the fate of Zosimus, Aristides was reluctant to obey these orders. In the end he solved the problem by sacrificing not a cow – which was forbidden – but a bull, and Asclepius was content.

The physicians were interested in Aristides' manifold divine apparitions. The reason they looked after him was partly out of fear that his health would deteriorate, but partly also out of scientific curiosity (2.20). Aristides mentions a physician by name of Heracleon, who was concerned about him as a friend, because he feared that he would become even more ill following an apparition he had at Smyrna. The condition Heracleon was concerned about was opisthotonus (spasms of the neck muscles). Yet in this case, too, all turned out well: Asclepius was again able to free Aristides of his affliction. Aristides referred to the ailment, which had worried his medical friend, Heracleon, so much, at a time (3.15–20) when he was already suffering from fever. An almost indescribable and unimaginable struggle had ensued. His body was torn in all directions, his knee pulled up against his head, his hands wildly flailing against his neck and face. His chest arched forward and his back pulled the opposite way so that Aristides likened his back to a sail inflated by the wind. After an extended stay at Pergamum the condition improved noticeably. Aristides general state of health improved after 147 CE, but he remained faithful to Asclepius, returning regularly to Pergamum for therapy and sacrifice. This, he thought, was the reason why he was spared when a plague (2.37–45) was rampant in the country in 165 CE (2.39 f., AMM. MARC. 23.6.24, LO CASCIO 2012, and GILLIAM 1961). Almost the entire neighbourhood was affected by this epidemic, first the servants and then he himself contracted it and suffered severely (2.39). Again it was Asclepius who appeared to him in a dream and healed him (SCHRÖDER 1988: 376).

Aristides was an eminent rhetorician whose great ambition was to make his mark on posterity. His claim in the *hieroi logoi* to write no less than three hundred thousand lines (2.3) and his immense diligence in composing this work (1.60) reveal the great enthusiasm he brought to this task (SCHRÖDER 1988: 376). He categorically refused the public office and duties specified in Antoninus Pius' decree for orators (DIG. 27.1.6.2 ff.). Freedom from the τέλη (*tele*), from personal duties (taking on offices, providing services) is referred to as ἀτέλεια (*ateleia*), which means exemption from taxes and financial obligations. This privilege was granted as a special honour to certain individuals. The condition was that they must not neglect their work. Aristides failed to meet this condition, or rather, he – just like the Gallic orator Flavorinus from Arelate (Arles) – was unwilling to meet it (PHILOSTR. soph. 480 and MEYER-ZWIFFELHOFER 2002: 124–127). Gaius Iulius Severus, who was proconsul of Asia at the time (152/153 CE), explained the dilemma most concisely (4.87):

ἀλλ᾽ ἕτερόν ἐστι πρῶτον ἑλλήνων εἶναι καὶ ἄκρον ἐν λόγοις – οὕτω γὰρ ὠνόμασεν – καὶ ἕτερον διατρίβειν ἐπὶ τούτῳ καὶ μαθητὰς ἔχειν.
It is one thing being the first of the Hellenes and an accomplished master of oratory (…) and another to do this in a professional way and have pupils.

Aristides' name was put forward for a number of public offices, an honour he – often quite vehemently – tried to reject. Severus proposed him for the office of peacekeeper (4.72); his name was also put forward for the post of *prytanis* (4.88); when Pollio was proconsul in Asia, he was appointed as tax collector (4.95); the citizens of Smyrna wanted to make him ἀρχιερεύς (*archiereus*) (4.101), or high priest, and give him the responsibility for the ceremony of the imperial cult. These appointments caused a veritable fight on Aristides' part to be released from any such honours. In the end he won thanks to the support he received from a friend, Gaius Iulius Quadratus Bassus, who was proconsul in 153/154 CE and who, shortly after taking up office, granted Aristides the privilege of *ateleia*.

After spending several years at Pergamum in search of a cure, Aristides had become a well-known orator and revered celebrity (4.71–108 and BEHR 1968: 41 ff.). According to Aristides' own words Asclepius himself emphasized his uniqueness as a speaker, when, upon being addressed by Aristides in the temple at Pergamum with the cultic formula "(You the) One," Asclepius responded with the words "You are (the One)" (4.50 and SCHRÖDER 1986: 100 note 129). Aristides expressed his gratitude for being thus honoured by composing a eulogy to Asclepius. The physicians also revered Aristides as a speaker. One of them, Porphyrius, is said to have stepped before the Cyzicans and promoted Aristides as a speaker (5.12). They received his speech with great enthusiasm. On his way to Ephesus, where Asclepius had sent him to speak in 170 CE, people showed immense interest in him – in his speech as much as in the baths he took there (2.81). He was held in high esteem even by Asclepius himself (4.13). In the fall of 170 CE Aristides described his physical condition, saying that he felt lighter and more cheerful than he had not done since his illness first started (5.48). The six consecutive months he spent in Cyzicus were the most productive of his entire career: they belonged to the period when Aristides lived in close proximity to Asclepius (6.1).

Analysis of the *hieroi logoi* reveals the general aspects that may be important for a patient-oriented historiography: Aristides reflects at length on himself and his body, dwelling on his feelings and experiences. He was sick and left extensive and detailed descriptions of his ailments. We learn much about his feelings over the years, his inner experience of his physical suffering, but also about his search for therapies and the effects these therapies had on his person and inner life. He became a patient of Asclepius at Pergamum and recorded his impressions of the therapies he underwent, describing how they were carried out and how he experienced them. He reflected on his relationship with the healthcare and the various healers, remarking on the incapability of the physicians and Asclepius' supremacy over them as the god who had saved him. He also related how others – physicians in particular – dealt with the therapies proposed by Asclepius. Aristides' notes are invaluable in this respect: the physicians first contributed their own wisdom and offered resistance, as was to be expected, but then they also found ways of arranging themselves with the situation. As the following analyses will show, they knew how to accommodate a medicine that was not all that different from their own methods. Aristides' discourses are therefore in many respects a valuable source which can add precision to the picture we have of the medicine of Asclepius.

In addition to Aristides' self-reflections we also have accounts from other patients. While these reports are considerably shorter they also contain fewer fictitious components. They appear in the form of votive inscriptions and record medical recommendations from the practice of Asclepius. They are reflections of patients concerning the therapies they received and include information about their stay at the sanctuary and about the mode, and success, of the treatments they received. This textual material is, again, not very detailed. There are thank-offerings that often do not mention more than the name of the donor, the deity, and in some cases also the reason for seeking treatment and, rarely, the cause of the condition also. It is not often possible to derive convincing arguments from them. Two examples need to be mentioned nonetheless, because they provide more detail and are open to analysis. They are unique examples from the second century CE and will both together form the centre of the following analysis: the first inscription was commissioned, at the behest of Asclepius (III.5.2), by M. Iulius Apellas from Mylasa in the region of Caria in Asia Minor (IG IV² 1.126). Apellas was a patient of Asclepius at Epidaurus where he received a therapy that was informed by cultic elements as well as by medical considerations. The treatment clearly overlaps with the medical method documented in the contemporary specialist literature. The names of illnesses in ancient medicine cannot really be compared with modern medical views: these names in themselves, as well as their connotations, have changed profoundly through the centuries. Additionally, the modern and ancient nosological terminologies differ substantially because the former focuses mainly on the anatomical location and morphological specificity of the ailment while the latter applies the nosology of the particular clinic. But it is mostly safe to look at the symptoms and at components of the therapy as long as one keeps LEVEN's (1998) methodological comments on retrospective diagnostics in mind.

The second inscription is by Publius Aelius Theon from Rhodes (MÜLLER 1987), who sought out Asclepius in his practice at Pergamum and, after being cured from his ailments, devoted the offering as a sign of his gratitude and obligation (III.5.3). His inscription helps to delineate the treatments in the Asclepieion in greater depth and illustrates that the medical therapy provided at Pergamum was in no way second to the contemporary scientific medicine. Both inscriptions are evidence of the symbiosis mentioned above of cultic and medical approaches. Despite their singularity, both sources are of great value, if one considers that the arguments so far have also confirmed this symbiosis. There were also miracle reports – they have been discussed at length – which must not be missing from an overall evaluation. But a synopsis of the wide-spread material reveals without doubt – as has also emerged from the argumentation in chapter III.2 – that one can assume that the two fields – religious-cultic medicine and scientific medicine, were intimately interwoven. The following analysis of the two votive gifts will confirm this view and will serve to support and corroborate the initial thesis put forward here of an independent Asclepian medicine.

III.5.2 – M. Iulius Apellas at Epidaurus

M. Iulius Apellas found relief from his affliction in the Asclepieion at Epidaurus and expressed his gratitude to Asclepius in a large epigram narrating the patient's perspective of the therapeutic treatment received there. The inscription dates back to the second century CE (fig. 20, IG IV² 1.126 and HAHN 1976). Because of its completeness it has become an object of investigation for various scientific disciplines. WILAMOWITZ (1886) and BAUNACK (1895) discerned similarities with the discourses of Aristides. KAVVADIAS (1900/1893/1885/1883), who was involved with the excavations carried out by the Greek Archaeological Society at Epidaurus, conceded that the content was rational to a degree as the excavations proceeded. HERZOG (1931) emphasized its psychological elements. EDELSTEIN/EDELSTEIN (1945) focused more on the medical aspects. MEIER (1967) cited Apellas as a witness of the interdependence of incubation and modern psychotherapy. RÜTTIMANN (1986: 46f.) made recourse again to Apellas' epigram, interpreting it however purely from the point of view of religious history, without paying any attention to medical considerations. The present investigation looks at Apellas' epigram in the light of the initial questions of the history of patients. It is therefore mainly concerned with the therapies at the Asclepieion from the perspective of Apellas, the patient. Apellas' donation is seen as an introspective testimonial of one of Asclepius' patients who received treatment in the Asclepieion in the second century CE and then provided information on his experience. Adopting this new methodical approach makes it legitimate to again make recourse to this much-investigated inscription which has become an authoritative example of Asclepian medicine.

ἐπὶ ἱερέως Πο(πλίου) Αἰλ(ίου) Ἀντιόχου
Μ(ᾶρκος) Ἰούλιος Ἀπελλᾶς Ἰδριεὺς Μυλασεὺς μετεπέμφθην
ὑπὸ τοῦ θεοῦ, πολλάκις εἰς νόσους ἐνπίπτων καὶ ἀπεψί-
αις χρώμενος. κατὰ δὴ τὸν πλοῦν ἐν Αἰγείνῃ ἐκέλευσέν
με μὴ πολλὰ ὀργίζεσθαι. ἐπεὶ δὲ ἐγενόμην ἐν τῷ ἱερῷ, ἐ-
κέλευσεν ἐπὶ δύο ἡμέρας συνκαλύψασθαι τὴν κεφαλήν,
ἐν αἷς ὄμβροι ἐγένοντο, τυρὸν καὶ ἄρτον προλαβεῖν, σέλει-
να μετὰ θρίδακος, αὐτὸν δι' αὑτοῦ λοῦσθαι, δρόμῳ, γυμνάζε-
σθαι, κιτρίου προλαμβάνειν τὰ ἄκρα, εἰς ὕδωρ ἀποβρέξαι, πρὸς
ταῖς ἀκοαῖς ἐν βαλανείῳ προστρίβεσθαι τῷ τοίχωι, περιπάτῳ χρῆ-
σθαι ὑπερῴῳ, αἰώραις, ἁφῇ πηλώσασθαι, ἀνυπόδητον περι-
πατεῖν, πρὶν ἐνβῆναι ἐν τῶι βαλανείῳ εἰς τὸ θερμὸν ὕδωρ
οἶνον περιχέασθαι, μόνον λούσασθαι καὶ Ἀττικὴν δοῦναι
τῶι βαλανεῖ, κοινῇ θῦσαι Ἀσκληπιῷ, Ἠπιόνῃ, Ἐλευσεινίαις,
γάλα μετὰ μέλιτος προλαβεῖν· μιᾷ δὲ ἡμέρᾳ πιόντός μου γάλα μόνον, εἶπεν· »μέλι ἔμβαλλε εἰς τὸ γάλα, ἵνα δύνηται διακό-
πτειν.« ἐπεὶ δὲ ἐδεήθην τοῦ θεοῦ θᾶττόν με ἀπολῦσαι, ᾤμην <ν>ά-
πυϊ καὶ ἁλσὶν κεχριμένος ὅλος ἐξιέναι κατὰ τὰς ἀκοὰς ἐκ τοῦ
ἀβάτου, παιδάριον δὲ ἡγεῖσθαι θυμιατήριον ἔχον ἀτμίζον
καὶ τὸν ἱερέα λέγειν »τεθεράπευσαι, χρὴ δὲ ἀποδιδόναι τὰ ἴατρα.«
καὶ ἐποίησα, ἃ εἶδον, καὶ χρειμένος μὲν τοῖς ἁλσὶ καὶ τῶι νάπυ-
ϊ ὑγρῶι ἤλγησα, λούμενος δὲ οὐκ ἤλγησα. ταῦτα ἐν ἐννέα ἡμέ-
ραις ἀφ' οὗ ἦλθον. ἥψατο δέ μου καὶ τῆς δεξιᾶς χιρὸς καὶ τοῦ
μαστοῦ, τῇ δὲ ἑξῆς ἡμέρᾳ ἐπιθύοντός μου φλὸξ ἀναδραμοῦ-
σα ἐπέφλευσε τὴν χεῖρα, ὡς καὶ φλυκταίνας ἐξανθῆσαι· μετ' ὀ-
λίγον δὲ ὑγιὴς ἡ χεὶρ ἐγένετο. ἐπιμείναντί μοι ἄνηθον με-
τ' ἐλαίου χρήσασθαι πρὸς τὴν κεφαλαλγίαν εἶπεν. οὐ μὴν ἤλ-
γουν τὴν κεφαλήν. συνέβη οὖν φιλολογήσαντί μοι συνπλη-
ρωθῆναι· χρησάμενος τῷ ἐλαίῳ ἀπηλλάγην τῆς κεφαλαλγί-
ας. ἀναγαργαρίζεσθαι ψυχρῷ πρὸς τὴν σταφυλὴν – καὶ γὰρ περὶ
τούτου παρεκάλεσα τὸν θεὸν – τὸ αὐτὸ καὶ πρὸς παρίσθμια. ἐκέ-
λευσεν δὲ καὶ ἀναγράψαι ταῦτα. χάριν εἰδὼς καὶ ὑγιὴς γε-
νόμενος ἀπηλλάγην.

In the priesthood of Publius Aelius Antiochus

I, Marcus Iulius Apellas, an Idrian from Mylasa, was sent for by the god,

For I was often ill and suffering from dyspepsia.

In the course of my journey, in Aegina, the god told me not to be so irritable.

When I arrived at the temple, he told me for two days to keep my head covered,

And for these two days it rained;

To eat cheese and bread, celery with lettuce,

To wash myself without help, to practise running,

To take lemon peels, to soak them in water,

near the (spot of the) *akoai* in the bath to press against the wall,

to take a walk in the upper portico,

to use the trapeze,

to rub myself with sand, to walk around barefoot,

in the bathroom, before plunging into the hot water, to pour wine over myself,

to bathe without help and to give an Attic drachma to the bath attendant,

in common to offer sacrifice to Asclepius, Epione and the Eleusinian goddesses,

to take milk with honey.

When one day I drank milk alone he said, "Put honey in the milk so that it can get through."

When I asked of the god to relieve me more quickly I thought I walked out of the abaton

Near the (spot of the) akoai, being anointed all over with mustard and salt,

While a small boy was leading me holding a smoking censer, and the priest said,

"You are cured but you must pay the thank-offerings."

And I did what I had seen, and when I anointed myself with the salts and the moistened mustard

I felt pain, but when I bathed I had no pain.

That happened within nine days after I had come.

He touched my right hand and also my breast.

The following day as I was offering sacrifice the flame leapt up and scorched my hand,

So that blisters appeared. Yet after a little, my hand was well again.

As I stayed on he said I should use dill and olive oil against my headaches.

I did not usually suffer from headaches.

But after I had studied, my head was congested.

After I used the olive oil the headache went away.

To gargle with a cold gargle for the uvula –

Since about that too I had consulted the god –

And the same also for the tonsils.

He bade me also inscribe this. Full of gratitude I departed well.

Apellas travelled to the Asclepieion at Epidaurus from Mylasa in Caria. Because of poor health – Apellas was often unwell with indigestion – the God had called him to his sanctuary. During his stay there Apellas heeded the instructions he received from Asclepius, hoping they would cure him. This turned out to be worthwhile because he was in good health again when he left the sanctuary.

Even on his way to the sanctuary, Apellas was asked by Asclepius to remain calm: possibly an indication of the patient's frail emotional state. In addition to the polymorbidity indicated – apart from hints at his susceptibility to illness and a digestive disorder, we find out from the epigram that Apellas contracted other illnesses during his stay – he was also mentally frail. What Apellas does not communicate is whether the new afflictions he acquired were a result of the therapies prescribed by Asclepius. The therapies proposed to Apellas illustrate the duality of medical therapy and cultic aspirations that is so typical of Asclepian medicine (EDELSTEIN/EDELSTEIN 1945: 139 and HAHN 1976: 49). The instruction to keep his head covered for two days is certainly not part of a medical therapy but rather of the mystery cult practised at the sanctuary. The cultic element is also reflected in the fact that Apellas was called to the sanctuary by Asclepius (WEINREICH 1909: 112 and MEIER 1967: 62). The patient from Caria leaves no doubt that his stay was initiated by Asclepius. The cultic aspects described run parallel to the medical-therapeutic instructions Apellas received from Asclepius, namely to wash without help and press against the wall at the *akoai*. What exactly the term ἀκοαί implies remains unclear (HAHN 1976: 27–29). The rubbing and massaging of body parts can have a relaxing as well as a soothing effect. At the same time these acts, as well as that of cleansing, are also important cultic rituals. Bodily cleanliness was expected of anyone entering the temple and water pools were therefore provided in the appropriate places in the sanctuaries (see chapter III.2). Apellas' description is paradigmatic of the concurrence of medical-therapeutic instructions and cultic-ritual provisions. Apellas mentions another cleansing ritual later, when he talks about being asked to pour wine over himself before entering the warm water; similarly with the instruction to walk barefoot, because being barefoot was an intrinsic part of initiation and lustration rituals. Apellas is, moreover, advised to apply sand to his body and take a warm bath. Warm baths were often used against weakness and inertia, but particularly also for the kind of sluggish digestion Apellas was afflicted with. Sand, too, was used as an effective, warming and healing, remedy. Water, like sand, has an additional cultic significance (STEGER 2005b). Apellas followed the instructions he received from Asclepius. His hope to be relieved from his ailments induced

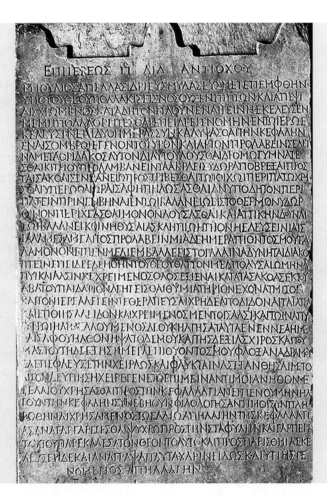

Fig. 20 – Inscription
by M. Iulius Apellas
from Mylasa in Caria
(IG IV² 1.126)

him to observe the medical-therapeutic as well as the cultic-ritual instructions given to him at the Asclepieion.

In addition, Apellas adhered to the following four therapeutic steps prescribed by Asclepius: the first was diet-related and consisted of fibre-rich food such as celery and lettuce, taken with plenty of fluids, mostly milk with honey. On two days Apellas was given cheese, bread, celery and lettuce. Bread was a common staple and formed the basis of every meal. According to the views held at the time cheese was considered more effective than milk for digestive disorders: if the stomach was affected, a mature cheese was used, grated and mixed with flour, if the problem was ileum-related a mild cheese was considered preferable. In case of colic a mixture of cheese and wine in a 1:3 ratio was recommended (PLIN. nat. 28.207; 20.140 and GAL. De san. Tuenda 6.696 K.).

In opposition to this, the Hippocratic Corpus suggests that cheese, whilst being nutritious, was the cause of constipation and bloating, indigestion and headaches (HIPPOKR. Vict. 2.51 (6.554.3–6 L.)). Lettuce is recommended for its cooling properties, in combination with celery, for instance. It refreshes, stimulates the appetite and, according to Galen and Pliny, also has a libido-reducing effect.

> (…) τὰ γε μὴν σέλινα καὶ τὰ σμύρνια καὶ τῆς θρίδακος φύλλοις μιγνύντες προσφέρονταί τινες. ἄποιον γὰρ οὖσα ἄχαον ἡ θρίδαξ, ἔτι τε ψυχρὸν ἔχουσα χυμὸν ἡδίων τε ἅμα καὶ ὠφελιμωτέρα γίνεται τῶν δριμέων τι προλαμβάνουσα (…).
>
> (…) some eat certainly celery and another plant with seeds that taste of myrrh, together with lettuce leaves. For lettuce which has no flavour of its own and, moreover, contains a cold juice, becomes more pleasant and more useful than spicier foods (…). (GAL. De alim. facult. 6.638.4–8 K.)

Unlike Galen, PLINY (nat. 19.127) differentiates between different kinds of lettuce:

> Purpuream maximae radicis Caecilianam vocant, rotundam vero ac minima radice, latis foliis ἀστυτίδα quidamque εὐνουχεῖον, quoniam haec maxime refragetur venari. Est quidem natura omnibus refrigeratrix et ideo aestate gratia. Stomacho fastidium auferunt cibique adpetentiam faciunt.

The purple lettuce with large roots is called "Caecilian," but the round lettuce with very small roots and broad leaves "astydis," sometimes "eunucheion" because it mostly reduces the libido. All of them have a cooling effect and are therefore pleasant in the summer. They remove the stomach's distaste for food and promote appetite.

Even in the Hippocratic Corpus we find indications both of the cooling properties of lettuce and its weakening effect on the body, while it is also recommended for burns and some women's disorders (HIPPOKR. Vict. 2.54 (6.558, 11 f. L.), Morb. Mul. 1,78 (8,196,10 L.) and 1.101 (8.224.16 f. L.)). Celery is said to promote diuresis (GAL. De alim. facult. 6.637 K.); the Hippocratic corpus mentions mostly the celery root for this purpose (HIPPOKR. Vict. 2.54 (6.558.13 f. L.)). Milk, like bread, is a common staple. Mixing milk with honey is known to have a soothing effect on the soul and relieve constipation. Any undigested intestinal contents will be moved on by this mixture. Honey is digested faster than any other foods and is therefore said to promote digestion if it is mixed with milk and appropriately dosed (GAL. De alim. facult. 6.685 K.).

According to the Hippocratic Corpus honey is nutritious in combination with other substances and gives a good complexion. Taken by itself it is said to have a weakening and strongly laxative effect. Goat's and ass's milk are also recommended for their laxative properties (HIPPOKR. Vict. 2.41 (6.538.17–20 L.)). In addition to following the dietetic instructions Apellas also takes the medicines prescribed by Asclepius, such as soaked lemon peel. GALEN points out that lemon, if a particular extract is prepared, promotes digestion (De alim. facult. 6.618 K.), while no specific properties are attributed to lemons in the Hippocratic Corpus. Together with honey, lemons promote the further processing of any bolus left behind in the gastro-intestinal tract.

With his thank-offering Apellas has left a therapy report that includes all the instructions he received. These therapeutic recommendations are, as comparison has revealed, in keeping with the contemporary medical views expressed in the specialist literature. It can be assumed that the therapeutic recommendations mentioned in the epigram arose from the prevalent medical thinking. Apellas is also told to gargle because of his swollen uvula. The instruction to use cold water is a reference to the general significance of cold-water treatments (HAHN 1976: 33). Apellas reports further how anointing himself with salt and mustard caused him pain. Salt has a cauterizing, burning and cleansing effect and was therefore often used in ointments prescribed against fatigue. Alongside mustard it has also been used in chemical peelings (URSIN/STEGER/BORELLI 2018). GALEN speaks of salt in connection with plasters (De comp. med. per gen. 13.504 K., 13.928 K. and 13.942 K.). Of all the medical traditions (II.3) it was the Methodists who assigned an irritating and inflammatory effect to mustard plasters (HAHN 1976: 38 f.). Apellas soon got rid of this particular pain by applying water. He also followed the advice to use dill and oil against his headache. The relief he soon experienced was mostly due to the cooling and therefore alleviating effect of the substances. GALEN spoke of dill as diuretic, analgesic and sleep-inducing (De dign. ex insomn. 6.832 K.). In the Hippocratic Corpus the herb is mentioned as a remedy against diarrhoea and sneezing (HIPPOKR. Vict. 2.54 (6.558.12 f. L.). External applications are not mentioned.

In addition to diets and medicines Apellas is also advised to take up physical exercise: he needed a recreational sport and was told to run and take walks. The attempt to explain the adjective ὑπερῷος as referring to withdrawing to a high altitude has quite rightly been rejected as absurd (HAHN 1976: 55). The final and last recommendation Apellas receives is to use the trapeze. Using the trapeze is seen as a form of relaxation: Apellas who suffered from persistent constipation needed to let go of any tension, which is also why he was advised at the very beginning of his journey to remain calm. Asclepius emphasized the need for Apellas to remain calm. His concept appears to have been successful since Apellas, after being subjectively cured of his afflictions at Epidaurus, left this gift as an expression of his gratitude and as a way of giving an account of his cure. His chronic constipation and any new disorders he contracted were treated with a therapy that consisted of dietary measures, medicines, light exercise and as much peace and rest as possible.

The therapy Apellas received was based on the contemporary medical thinking and included also components such as exercise and rest, which are familiar to us from modern health spas. This approach can be seen as specific to Asclepian medicine. The account left by Apellas is evidence of a therapeutic method that was customary in the Asclepieia. This testimonial constitutes a further argument in support of the thesis that Asclepian medicine was an independent approach which can only be fully understood in its complexity if the diverse sources are being consulted. That this method was not purely a healing cult is confirmed by the account left by Apellas.

III.5.3 – P. Aelius Theon at Pergamum

Another therapy report from the second century CE was left by one P. Aelius Theon who spent time at the sanctuary at Pergamum (MÜLLER 1987). The dating of this source is supported paleographically, by the fact of Hadrian's ascension to the throne in 117 CE as a *terminus post quem*, and by the fact that it was customary to mention both the *praenomen* and *nomen* of new Roman citizens, in this case: Publius Aelius Theon. Another votive from Pergamum by the same dedicant, which refers to an altar of Eurostia, also goes back to the second century CE (IvP III 127 and MÜLLER 1987: 198). Theon, too, gives a patient's point of view of the therapies he received.

Ἀσκληπιῶι φιλανθρώπωι· θεῶι Πό(πλιος) Αἴλ(ιος)
Θέων Ζηνοδότου καὶ Ζηνοδό[τ]ης Ῥόδιος
ἑκατὸν εἴκοσι ἡμερῶν μὴ πιὼν καὶ φαγὼν ἔωθεν ἑκάστης ἡμέρας λευκοῦ πι-
πέπερος κόκκους δεκαπέντε καὶ κρομμύου
[ἥ]μισυ κατὰ κέλευσιν τοῦ θεοῦ ἐναργῶς ἐκ
[πολ]λῶν καὶ μεγάλων κινδύνων σωθεὶς
[ἀνέ]θηκα καὶ ὑπὲρ τοῦ ἀδελφιδοῦ Πο(πλίου) Αἰλ(ίου)
[Καλλι]στράτου τοῦ καὶ Πλαγκιανοῦ. vac.
[ἀντιπ]άτρου τὸ παιδικὸν εὐχήν. vac.

To Asclepius, the god who loves humankind, I, Publius Aelius Theon – son of Ze-
nodotus and Zenodote from Rhodes, who, for 120 days, did not drink and, in the
early morning of each day, ate fifteen grains of white pepper and half an onion, as
recommended by the God, and was manifestly saved from many great dangers –
have dedicated, also on behalf of my nephew Publius Aelius Callistratus, who is also
called Plancianus, the son of Antipater, the παιδικὸν according to his vow.

The inscription speaks of the dedication of Publius Aelius Theon, who devoted
a παιδικόν (*paidikon*) to the philanthropic Asclepius, on the one hand to thank
him for the diet he prescribed and on the other because of a vow made by
his nephew, a certain Publius Callistratus. This inscription is obviously much
shorter than the one dedicated by Apellas, and it contains fewer statements
which are suitable for medical evaluation. Theon's inscription merely mentions Asclepius' dietary recommendation to eat fifteen white peppercorns and
half an onion in the mornings (on an empty stomach), that Theon adhered
to this diet for 120 days and that the therapy was successful. Theon refers to
Asclepius as a φιλάνθρωπος (philanthrope) and, like Apellas and Aristides, he
emphasizes his good relationship with the god.

Theon received his dietary instructions κατὰ κέλευσιν τοῦ θεοῦ (on order of the God), which means that Asclepius appeared to him in his dream
and imparted his recommendations. Incubation, which can be described as
a transitional ritual, was the most characteristic therapeutic measure applied
in the Asclepieia. Theon's epigram confirms the incubation process from the
point of view of the patient: Theon received his prescriptions in a dream.
WEINREICH (1909: V–VIII) pointed out in this context that, aside from the
miraculous dream healings, one had to differentiate between healing through
images and healing by the holy hand. We have already explained in some detail the necessity to distinguish between dream healings in the actual sense of
the word, which are known mostly from Christian miracle reports, and the
healings where instructions are conveyed in a dream, as in the present example (DODDS 1970: 55–71). The instructions Theon received from Asclepius in
his dream, saved him from numerous serious dangers. He was probably referring to complications resulting from his illness. Theon writes that the god
helped him "manifestly" (ἐναργῶς), which seems to indicate that the therapy
of Asclepius was successful. ἐναργεία describes the God's faculty of transcend-
ence that elevates him above human rationality and understanding. Attempts
have been made time and again to derive some miraculous element from this
(MÜLLER 1987: 205); but the term has also been used by other delighted dev-

otees who sought to express their gratitude. The epigram documents a dream prescription not a miraculous act.

Out of gratitude for his successful cure, Theon dedicated a *paidikon* to Asclepius. It has not been possible to determine exactly what this votive gift entailed. MÜLLER (1987: 205) states quite rightly that it will hardly refer to the Platonic 'pleasure boy' mentioned in the *Symposion*. Theon dedicates this unidentifiable *paidikon* not only to give expression to his gratitude, as he himself explains, but also on behalf of his nephew, Publius Aelius Callistratus. An inscription from Lindos testifies that Theon was cured by Asclepius while his nephew Callistratus died at a young age. The gift is therefore given partly in thankfulness for himself and partly in reverent commemoration of his nephew Callistratus who died young (BLINKENBERG 1917: 465).

The short inscription, although self-reflective in character, does not allow for conclusions regarding Theon's illness, but one can indirectly try to derive from it information as to the nature of his affliction and conclude that he suffered from a digestive problem (MÜLLER 1987: 218). Asclepius prescribes a 120-day therapy for Theon, which consists in his eating fifteen white pepper corns and half an onion early every morning (on an empty stomach). As in the case of Apellas, we can again understand and explain the therapies suggested if we refer to the medical ideas transmitted in the contemporary specialist literature.

Two natural remedies are mentioned: pepper and onion. GALEN ascribed a warming effect to onions (In Hipp. Epid. VI comment. 17.2.285 K.) and therefore thought them harmful for a warm stomach:

> (...) κρόμμυα δηλονότι καὶ σκόροδα καὶ σίλφιον καὶ ὀπὸν οἶνόν τε παλαιότατον ὅσα τ᾽ ἄλλα
> τοιαῦτα τὴν φυσικὴν δυσκηκφασίαν αὐξάντα, τῆ· δὲ ταυτῆς ἐναντία χρησιμώτατα (...).
> (...) Onions, garlic, silphium, the juice of the fig tree and very old wine – they all promote the development of a bad temperament and everything that works against this is extremely useful (...).

That onions are harmful to a warm stomach had already been stated in the Hippocratic Corpus. Onion is bad for the body because it causes excessive warmth (HIPPOKR. Aff. 54 (6.264.12 f. L.)). It was used for digestive disorders because of its bloating effect (CELS. artes 2.26.1, DIOSC. mat. med. 2.151.1 and PLIN. nat. 20.42 f.). Pepper also has a warming effect (GAL. De temper. 1.682 K., De simpl. medicament. temp. 11.421 K.). The Hippocratic Corpus, too, recommends pepper for various afflictions: stitches in the side, directly after they occur (HIPPOKR. Acut. 11 (2.466.2 L.), to facilitate expectoration in chest infections, and in combination with chicken broth against tetanus (Morb. 3.12 (7.132.12–14 L.). Toothache sufferers are advised to rinse their mouth with pepper and castoreum (HIPPOKR. Epid. 5.67 (5.244.7 f. L.)). Lastly, an "Indian Mixture" made up of aniseed, dill, myrrh, pepper and wine is recommended for the cleaning of teeth (HIPPOKR. Mor. Mul. 2.205 (8.394.8–10 L.)). The effect of pepper and onion therefore lies in their joint generation of warmth and they were used accordingly: their warming power was diuretic as well as digestive (CELS. artes 2.27; 2.31; 2.19,1, DIOSC. mat. med. 2.159.3, CELS. artes 2.19.1, and GAL. De san. tuenda 6.340 f. K.), and their combined use was also recommended to combat lethargy (CELS. artes 3.20.1).

Lastly, we will look at two details of this inscription which are discussed by scholars (MÜLLER 1987: 219 f.): one of them concerns the exact mode of application, the other the question as to whether the instruction to Publius Aelius Theon to refrain from drinking for 120 days referred to mornings only or to the whole day. The order given by Asclepius advised Theon to take the pepper and onion on an empty stomach so that these natural remedies could unfold their optimal effect and because the organism was then better able to absorb them. The few lines contained in this inscription clearly mention an empty stomach in the morning: "ἑκατὸν εἴκοσι ἡμερῶν μὴ πιὼν καὶ φαγὼν ἔωθεν ἑκάστης ἡμέρας" ("[who] for 120 days did not drink or eat in the early morning.) MÜLLER's discussion (1987: 222) as to whether, if one included GALEN's radical non-drinking theory (GAL. Syn. libr. de puls. 9.488 K. and GAL. In Hipp. Acut. comment. 15.498–501 K.; 15.575–577 K.; 15.695 K. and also 15.700–704 K.), this instruction could be interpreted as meaning to remain without food all day long is meaningless because the text is unambiguous in this respect. From a linguistic point of view, the passage clearly refers to fasting in the morning. Reading this text as meaning that not drinking was a typical measure used in the Pergamene Asclepieion would be absurd. The intrinsic scientific problem that is concealed behind this kind of argument becomes apparent when one deals with such healing reports. It is not simply a matter of correcting erroneous thinking, but one needs to raise awareness of a problem in the history of research and of science that manifests particularly in the evaluation of accounts of cures.

Additionally, it is of interest to the historian of economy that pepper was very expensive and therefore not affordable for everyone. Pepper (*P. album et P. nigrum*) was a precious spice which was imported from India and which had gained growing importance in the imperial period. The inscription discussed earlier mentioned that Apellas had to pay the bath attendant an Attic drachma. Both the pepper and the drachma, in conjunction, corroborate the thesis put forward in chapter III.2 that the larger sanctuaries of the imperial period, which included medical and cultic elements, a theatre, sports facilities and libraries, grew to be places where the members of the rich upper classes gathered.

The votive gift left by Theon transmits a healing report which, although it is shorter and yields only scarce medical information, conveys therapeutic prescriptions similar to Apellas' testimony of Epidaurus which are much more than mere cultic directions. Comparing these prescriptions with the medical ideas expressed in the contemporary specialist literature provides proof, in both Theon's and Apellas' case, that the therapeutic recommendations arose from the medical thinking of the time and that they were rational.

Taken together, the healing reports of Apellas and of Theon, the impressions left by Aristides and the results of the architectural analysis of the Asclepian sanctuaries in chapter III.2 leave no doubt that, in his sanctuaries, Asclepius provided a complex combination of therapies, in which medicine played an important part. It is true, and this has been pointed out in the first part of this chapter, that the testimonies documenting the cultic-medical aspirations of the Asclepian cult are mostly epigraphic. Since the second century CE, due to the growing rivalry with Christianity, these testimonies have been dominated by reports of miraculous cures. Such reports made it possible to emphasize the divine power behind these cures and for Asclepius Soter to compete with Christ Soter. But – and the various analyses have been able to show this convincingly – the admittedly sparse sources do yield, aside from cultic information, also medical insights that are in keeping with the contemporary specialist literature:

The medicine of Asclepius, as performed in the Asclepieia, is characterized by its two aspects, which come together in a meaningful way. They are not in contradiction to each other, because it is the very interweaving of the medical therapies and the cultic-ritual acts that makes this form of medicine what it is: the medicine of Asclepius, which constitutes one piece in the huge mosaic of the health and healer market described in chapter II.

IV

Summary

The myth of Asclepius and his healing cult have been scrutinized by researchers from a multitude of aspects (I). The work done so far has largely been conducted from the point of view of religious history and little attention has been given to medical questions. In the present investigation the attempt is made to remedy this situation by examining the medicine of Asclepius during the Roman Empire in close detail and integrating it into the highly differentiated healthcare market of the time.

It first introduces the multifarious agents on this healing market (II): the differentiated system which emerged during the imperial period grew from theoretical and practical medical foundations which were rooted in an earlier era. The cultural beginnings (II.1) of imperial healthcare go back far beyond ancient Greece. Asclepius, the hero and later god of healing, whose cult and, above all, whose medicine form the centre of this examination, is eminently suited to exemplify this wider cultural context. The connection between Asclepius and the ancient Babylonian healing deity Gula of Isin can be demonstrated on the basis of the fact that dogs played an important part in both healing cults. This link is one example of a wider cultural exchange between ancient Babylon and Hellas. It calls attention to the fact that the medical thinking and practice we meet in the imperial period arose from a variety of cultural impulses (STEGER 2004: 167–195). There is evidence that similar relationships existed between Asclepius and Imhotep (ŁAJTAR 2006), or Asclepius and Eshmun.

Medical practice and the endeavour to place this practice on theoretical foundations go hand in hand. The Ionian natural philosophers started this process when they prepared the ground for a medical theory in Rome. There is, however, no single – or even prominent – medical theory but rather a heterogeneous field in which the many diverse traditions each have a place (II.3): the Dogmatists continued the ancient tradition of medical rationalism, holding that illness had covert as well as overt causes. Therapies were in their view always based on conjecture. The Empiricists opposed the idea of covert causes and insisted that experience was all-important. The Methodists, who joined the Empiricists' in this criticism, adopted some of the ideas of Asclepiades of Bithynia and developed their own medical theory. They went on to become the central medical group in the imperial period. The Pneumatics thought that the *pneuma*, from which the world forms the human body, is manifest in the pulse. And lastly, there were the Anonymists whose ideas were based on humoral pathology. Next to these five traditions there were also individuals who established their own medical theories (II.4). We owe it to the literary activity of these individuals that their theories are still accessible. The first of these individuals we need to mention is Aretaeus of Cappadocia who flourished in the middle of the first century CE and whose work is close to the pneumatic tradition and to the writings of the Hippocratic Corpus. His contemporary Scribonius Largus was another important figure in the medical world: he composed a pharmacology that was also accessible to patients and that empowered them to choose their own healthcare provider. Pedanius Dioscorides of Anazarbus who, for part of his career, served as a military physician under Nero, attempted to found a new pharmacology which was suitable for lay-people as well as specialists. Rufus of Ephesus was a contemporary of Trajan who studied the principles of Hippocratic medicine with a critical eye. Aulus Cornelius Celsus, whose status as a physician is controversially discussed by scholars, has left an encyclopaedia of practical science. Galen of Pergamum's extensive opus on medical theory has a long and important history of reception. Galen, who did not descend from a family of physicians, made a name for himself as a medical practitioner to gladiators and at the imperial court. He did not subscribe to any of the philosophies or medical traditions but studied several approaches critically and developed his own direction. Galen's practical activity is particularly suited to illustrate the close connection between medical practice and the search for theoretical foundations.

Medical theory went hand in hand with the everyday medical practice (II.5) which benefitted from the transfer of medical thinking and actions. The *medicina domestica*, which demonstrably goes back to early Roman times and consisted in the treatment of family members and servants by the *paterfamilias*, was enriched by healing approaches ranging from magical-demonist to theurgic to the scientific-rational system that is based on the observation and understanding of nature. The group of scientific physicians alone can be divided into public, private and military practitioners. The public physicians, called ἀρχιατρός or *archiater*, are closest to our modern concept of medical practitioners. The ancient term ἰατρός or ἰατήρ, on the other hand, is much wider and cannot be clearly defined because specializations were wide-spread since the fourth century BCE and we have no evidence of any binding training guidelines or state examinations. The only rules we know of refer to the provision of medical services. Anyone who received instruction in τέχνη ἰατρική (the art of healing) could become a medical doctor so that the teacher, who among other things also conveyed the theoretical foundations, played a crucial part in specialist training. There was a wide array of medical practitioners. Physicians qualified in their profession by gaining experience and providing proof of their knowledge. Women also practised medicine. They were referred to as *medica* or ἰατρίνη. Scholars argue whether the term ἰατρίνη was used to refer to a midwife (μαῖα). There is evidence of female physicians who were experts in their profession but their sphere of work was usually restricted to the treatment of women and children. It is difficult to present the everyday medical activities of individual practitioners because there is generally very little information available. The evidence we do have is mostly of male public physicians. They were employed to look after the health of the general population in a town or city and received special favours or privileges in return. Some physicians practised at the imperial court, such as Antonius Musa who served the Emperor Augustus, and Gaius Stertinius Xenophon, who was first employed by Tiberius and later by Claudius. Generally, physicians had the same status as craftsmen. There was an unlimited number of practising private physicians who had to prove their practical skills and knowledge to an ever better informed population. While physicians had the status of craftsmen at the beginning of the imperial period, they grew steadily more prosperous from the second century CE onwards. The third group of medical practitioners, the military physicians, provided healthcare in the army alongside the medical orderlies and the veterinarians. This military medical service gained greater significance under Augustus. The physicians in question were either recruited for a fixed period of time or they took on more permanent positions offering their services in the sickrooms or *valetudinaria*. This system was in principle quite flexible, but a certain medical hierarchy was noticeable nevertheless. All three medical groups represented a medicine that claimed to be scientific and rational, in keeping with the contemporary specialist literature. Additionally, the healthcare market was enriched by non-medical groups that included masseurs, nurses, and the manufacturers and sellers of drugs and medicinal products. Another dimension of healthcare that is not to be underestimated is the whole range of magic and religious approaches (III.1): As we know from Egyptian papyri magic was applied in parallel with the combination of medicine, religion, and astrology in the attempt to combat illness. Magical-religious aspects of medicine are apparent in propitiatory inscriptions from the first to the third centuries CE in Asia Minor. These documents portray illness as the result of a sinful life and the confession of sins as prerequisite to healing.

Curing illnesses was the task of heroes and gods. The healing cult of Asclepius (III.1) stands out, not least due to the fact that, like the cults of Heracles and Serapis, it reached far beyond the Mediterranean world. According to the myth Apollo, the father of Asclepius, set the Greek people free from the plague, and Asclepius was so greatly concerned with people's health that he tried to extend their lives beyond the biological limit, an endeavour for which he was severely punished. Asclepius then became prominent in portrayals and in sanctuaries that were devoted to him alone where he was worshipped and where the sick came to be cured. The Asclepian cult first started in Epidaurus and spread out from there: in the fourth century BCE Pergamum and Cos were founded, and at the beginning of the third century BCE the cult arrived on Tiber Island in Rome. For the early first century BCE more than 300 cultic sites are documented for Asclepius. During the imperial period the Asclepian healing cult spread further and further, reaching a climax in the second century CE, thanks also to Hadrian and Antoninus Pius, under whose reigns the towns of Asia Minor saw an economic and cultural boom. Because the sanctuaries grew in size, the cult of Asclepius became more important and developed into a serious competitor of Christianity. The sanctuaries at Pergamum and at Aegeae in Cilicia enjoyed the patronage of Caracalla so that Asclepius and his cult retained their prominence even through the notorious "crisis" of the third century CE. Asclepius is the leading representative of the pagan healing cults; together with the emperor as healer he faces Christ the healer. In the dualism of Christianity and paganism, Asclepius and his healing cult were able to survive for a long time, not giving way to the Christian rival until the sixth century CE.

The patients of Asclepius received care in his sanctuaries. The social function of the architecture of the Asclepieia (III.2) is therefore also important in this context. This architecture, just like the medical practice, is part of the everyday medical culture: their location was chosen in accordance with the social and medical needs of the patients. A healthy position with beneficial springs was recommended (Epidaurus, Cos, Pergamum). The analysis of the architectural set-up of the sanctuaries follows the stations through which the devotees passed in the course of their therapies. It is important to note that the patients were accommodated separately, in buildings outside the temple precinct, as we can see from the sanctuary in Cos. Treatment did not take place in the residential buildings but only in the sanctuary. The argument that the Asclepieia were an early form of hospital is therefore not convincing. Contact between Asclepius and the devotee was established in the sanctuary, which included springs, pools and buildings containing fountains. Here, the devotees had the possibility to wash before entering the sanctuary in order to meet the requirement for purity. Any balneological components of the therapy prescribed were also administered here. Once the devotee had undergone the ritual preparation of cleansing, prayer and the offering of sacrifices, Asclepius would appear to him in the *abaton* (the sleeping quarters). The incubation can be described as a rite of passage. After his dream encounter with Asclepius the devotee would leave the sacred precinct and make thank-offerings to the god. The numerous devotional gifts that have been preserved reveal details of the healthcare received. The set-up of the sanctuaries was part of a holistic therapy concept that included libraries, theatres and sports facilities and offered patients a pleasant and restorative sojourn in a health-promoting ambience.

It is noticeable that only few self-reflective testimonials from patients of Asclepius have been preserved. When these patients left the sanctuary, they donated devotional gifts with inscriptions in which they expressed their gratitude to Asclepius (III.3). Some of them depict the body parts in question (anatomical votives), others give insight into the dreams. When it comes to these dream reports we need to make a distinction: on the one hand there are those that resemble the Christian miracle reports because they speak of miraculous healings which occurred in dreams. Such miracle healings were also used as propaganda to support the topos of "the emperor as healer" (Vespasian and Hadrian). On the other hand there are the reports that describe the therapies and the healthcare provided "from below", that is, from the patient's point of view. This new methodical access (III.4), which is favoured by the history of patients, gives insight into the outer and inner experiences of the patients. A very good example of this patient view was left by P. Aelius Aristides, who, after spending many years as a patient of Asclepius, gave interesting details of the Pergamene sanctuary in his *Sacred Tales* (III.5.1). At first glance, these ego-documents seem to offer reliable access to Aristides' own experience of his body and to his view of the therapies offered in the Pergamene Asclepieion. If one looks more closely at his narrative one finds that much of it can only be fiction. The way Aristides dealt with illness shows how he reflected on himself, his illnesses, and his experiences in the Asclepieia. He presents an impressive image of a patient of Asclepius at Pergamum, describes how his therapies unfolded and how he, as a patient, experienced the healthcare he received there. The writings of Aristides are highly valuable sources when it comes to the question of how others, physicians in particular, dealt with the therapies suggested by Asclepius. We learn for instance that the physicians managed to make compromises with the Asclepian medicine. Other imperial inscriptions referring to Asclepian therapies are far more concise: from Epidaurus a report has been transmitted by one M. Iulius Apellas from Mylasa in Caria (III.5.2), whom Asclepius healed of his afflictions and who expressed his gratitude by leaving this inscription. Close analysis of this therapy report reveals that the therapy prescribed for Apellas was based on the contemporary medical thinking and that it included measures which are characteristic of Asclepian medicine, such as exercise and rest, both of which are still part of healthcare regimes today. P. Aelius Theon also left an account of his stay at Pergamum (III.5.3). Like the first report mentioned, this one also includes cultic healing instructions but also therapies known from the medical tradition. Taken together, the analysis of the architectural set-up and of the patient reports prove without any doubt that the medicine of Asclepius in the imperial period included a complex fabric of therapies, in which medicine played an important part and which was informed by the interweaving of cultic-ritual practices and medical therapies. The medicine of Asclepius was therefore an independent medical approach that formed an important facet of the general health and healer market of the Roman Empire (II).

Appendix

V.1 – Editions and translations

For ancient authors the common scientific editions have been used. They are not listed separately. Authors and works are abbreviated according to Hubert CANCIK and Helmuth SCHNEIDER (ed.): Der Neue Pauly. Enzyklopädie der Antike. Vol. 1. Stuttgart, Weimar 1996, p. XXXIX–XLVII. Works from the Corpus Hippocraticum and Corpus Galenicum are cited according to FICHTNER (2017/2018).

Aelii Aristidi Smyrnaei quae supersunt omnia edidit Bruno KEIL (1948). Vol. II. Orationes XVII–LIII continens. Berlin.

ANONYM (1982): Der orphische Papyrus von Derveni. In: ZPE 47, Anhang, p. 1–12.

AULUS CORNELIUS Celsus (2016): De Medicina / Die medizinische Wissenschaft. 3 Vols. Edition, commentary and translation by Thomas Lederer. Darmstadt.

BORGER, Rykle (1982): Übersetzung des Codex Hammurapi. In: KAISER, Otto (ed.): Texte aus der Umwelt des Alten Testaments. Vol. 1. Rechtsbücher. Gütersloh.

Claudii Galeni opera omnia. 20 Vols. Edited by Carl G. KÜHN. Leipzig 1821–1833 (also Hildesheim 1965).

EDELSTEIN, Emma J.; EDELSTEIN, Ludwig (1945): Asclepius. A collection and interpretation of the testimonies. 2 Vols. Baltimore (also 1998 in one volume).

GIRONE, Maria (1998): Ἰάματα. Guarigioni miracolose di Asclepio in testi epigrafici. Test., introd., trad. e commento a cura di Maria Girone, con un contributo di Maria Totti-Gemünd. Bari.

GUARDUCCI, Margherita (1978): Epigrafia Greca IV. Epigrafi sacre pagane e christiane. Rom.

HABICHT, Christian (1969): Die Inschriften des Asklepieions von Pergamon (= Altertümer von Pergamon, VIII,3). Berlin.

HEINRICHS, Albert (1974): Papyri Graecae magicae. Die griechischen Zauberpapyri. Stuttgart.

KEARSLEY, Rosalinde A. (2001): Greeks and Romans in Imperial Asia. Mixed language inscriptions and linguistic evidence for cultural interaction until the end of AD III (= Inschriften griechischer Städte aus Kleinasien, 59). Bonn.

KLEIN, Richard (1983): Die Romrede des Aelius Aristides (= Texte zur Forschung, 45). Darmstadt.

LIDONNICI, Lynn R. (1995): The Epidaurean Miracle Inscriptions. Text, translation and commentary. Atlanta.

MÜRI, Walter (1979): Der Arzt im Altertum. Griechische und lateinische Quellenstücke von Hippokrates bis Galen mit der Übertragung ins Deutsche. 4. Auflage. München.

Œuvres complètes d'Hippocrate, traduction nouvelle avec le texte grec Émile LITTRÉ (1839–1861). 20 Vols. Paris (also Amsterdam 1961–1963 and 1973–1991).

PEEK, Werner (1963): Fünf Wundergeschichten aus dem Asklepieion von Epidauros. Berlin.

PETZL, Georg (1994): Die Beichtinschriften Westkleinasiens (= Epigraphica Anatolica, 22). Bonn.

PFOHL, Gerhard (1977): Inschriften der Griechen. Epigraphische Quellen zur Geschichte der antiken Medizin. Darmstadt.

PLEKET, Henri W. (1969): Epigraphica II. Texts on the Social History of the Greek World. Leiden.

Publius Aelius Aristides (1986): Heilige Berichte. Einleitung, deutsche Übersetzung und Kommentar von Heinrich O. SCHRÖDER, Vorwort von H. Hommel. Heidelberg.

P. Aelii Aristidis opera quae exstant omnia (1976): Volumen primum orations I – XVI complectens. Orationes I et V – XVI edidit Fridericus Waltharius LENZ, praefationem conscripsit et orationes II, III, IV edidit Carolus Allison BEHR. Leiden.

SCHUBERT, Charlotte; HUTTNER, Ulrich (ed.) (1999): Frauenmedizin in der Antike. Griechisch-lateinisch-deutsch (= Sammlung Tusculum). Düsseldorf, Zürich.

VENTRIS, Michael; CHADWICK, John (1973): Documents in Mycenaean Greek. 2nd edition. Cambridge.

VICTOR, Ulrich (1997): Lukian von Samostata: Alexandros oder der Lügenprophet (= Religions in the Graeco-Roman World, 132). Leiden, New York, Köln.

V.2 – Bibliography

A

AGELIDIS, Soi (2011): Kulte und Heiligtümer in Pergamon. In: GRÜSSINGER (2011), p. 174–183.

AHEARNE-KROLL, Stephen P. (2014): Mnemosyne at the Asklepieia. In: Classical Philology 109, p. 99–118.

ALBUTT, Thomas C. (1921): Greek Medicine in Rome. London.

ALESHIRE, Sara B. (1989): The Athenian Asklepieion. The people, their dedications and the invatories. Amsterdam.

ALESHIRE, Sara B. (1991): Asklepios at Athens. Epigraphic and prosopographic essays on the Athenian healing cults. Amsterdam.

ALLAN, Nigel (2001): The Physician in Ancient Israel: His Status and Function. In: Medical History 45, p. 377–394.

AMANDRY, Michel (1993): Un monnayage d'Hadrien à Èpidaure. In: Revue des études grecques 106, p. 329–333.

ASSMANN, Jan (2000): Weisheit und Mysterium. Das Bild der Griechen von Ägypten. München.

AUFFARTH, Christoph (1995): Aufnahme und Zurückweisung ‚Neuer Götter' im spätklassischen Athen: Religion gegen die Krise, Religion in der Krise? In: Eder, Walter (ed.): Die athenische Demokratie im 4. Jahrhundert v. Chr. Vollendung oder Verfall einer Verfassungsform? Stuttgart, p. 337–365.

AVALOS, Hector (1995): Illness and Health Care in the Ancient Near East. The role of the temple in Greece, Mesopotamia, and Israel (= Harvard Semitic Monographs, 54). Atlanta.

B

BAADER, Gerhard (1967): Spezialisierung in der Spätantike. In: Medizinhistorisches Journal 2, p. 231–238.

BAUNACK, Johannes (1895): Zu den Inschriften aus Epidauros. In: Philologus 54, p. 16–63.

BECHER, Ilse (1970): Antike Heilgötter und die römische Staatsreligion. In: Philologus 114, p. 211–255.

BEHR, Charles A. (1968): Aelius Aristides and the Sacred Tales. Amsterdam.

BEHR, Charles A. (1969): Aelius Aristides' Birth Date, corrected to November 29, 117 A. D. In: American Journal of Philology 90, p. 75–83.

BELOW, Karl-Heinz (1953): Der Arzt im römischen Recht (= Münchener Beiträge zur Papyrusforschung und antiken Rechtsgeschichte, 37). München.

BENEDUM, Christa (1990): Asklepios – Der homerische Arzt und der Gott von Epidauros. In: Rheinisches Museum 133, p. 210–226.

BENEDUM, Christa (1996): Der frühe Asklepios. In: Orbis Terrarum 2, p. 9–40.

BENEDUM, Jost (1977): Griechische Arztinschriften aus Kos. In: Zeitschrift für Papyrologie und Epigraphik 25, p. 272–274.

BESNIER, Maurice (1902): L'île Tibérine dans l'antiquité. Paris.

BIRABEN, Jean-Noel (1996): Das medizinische Denken und die Krankheiten in Europa. In: GRMEK (1996), p. 356–401.

BIRLEY, Anthony N. (1997): Caracalla. In: CLAUSS (1997a), p. 185–191.

BITTRICH, Ursula (2016): Traum. Mantik. Allegorie. Die „Hieroi Logoi" des Aelius Aristides im weiteren Kontext der griechisch-römischen Traumliteratur. (= Millennium-Studien / Millennium Studies). Berlin.

BLINKENBERG, Christian (1917): Lindiaka. Kobenhavn.

BLIQUEZ, Lawrence J. (2015): The tools of Asclepius. Surgical instruments in Greek and Roman times (= Studies in Ancient Medicine, 43). Leiden, Boston.

BLUMENBERG, Hans (1971): Wirklichkeitsbegriff und Wirkungspotential des Mythos. In: Fuhrmann, Manfred (ed.): Terror und Spiel. Probleme der Mythenrezeption (= Poetik und Hermeneutik, 4). München, p. 11–66.

BLUMENBERG, Hans (1979): Arbeit am Mythos. Frankfurt/M.

BRASHEAR, William M. (1995): The Greek Magical Papyri. An introduction and survey. Annotated bibliography. In: ANRW II 18,5. Berlin, New York, p. 3380–3684.

BREITWIESER, Rupert; HUMER, Franz; POLLHAMMER, Eduard; ARNOTT, Robert (2018): Medizin und Militär – Soldiers and Surgeons. Beiträge zur Wundversorgung und Verwundetenfürsorge im Altertum (Neue Forschungen / Archäologischer Park Carnuntum). St. Pölten.

BRODERSEN, Kai (ed.) (2015): Galenus: Die verbrannte Bibliothek. Peri alypias/Über die Unverdrossenheit. Wiesbaden.

BRUIT ZAIDMAN, Louise; SCHMITT PANTEL, Pauline (1994): Die Religion der Griechen. Kult und Mythos. München.

BÜHLER, Axel; COHNITZ, Daniel (2005): Ärzteschulen. In: LEVEN (2005), col. 15–16.

BÜYÜKKOLANCI, Mustafa; ENGELMANN, Helmut (1991): Inschriften aus Ephesos. In: Zeitschrift für Papyrologie und Epigraphik 86, p. 137–144.

BURFORD, Alison (1969): The Greek Temple Builders of Epidauros. Liverpool.

BURKERT, Walter (1972): Homo necans. Interpretationen altgriechischer Opferriten und Mythen. Berlin, New York.

BURKERT, Walter (1979): Structure and History in Greek Mythology and Ritual. Berkeley.

BURKERT, Walter (1984): Die orientalisierende Epoche in der griechischen Religion und Literatur. Heidelberg.

C

CASTRITIUS, Helmut (1973): Materiell-ökonomische Hintergründe der Christenverfolgungen im Römischen Reich. In: CASTRITIUS, Helmut; LOTTER, Friedrich; MEYER, Hermann; NEUHAUS, Helmut (ed.): Herrschaft, Gesellschaft, Wirtschaft. Vol. 1. Donauwörth, p. 82–95.

CAVANAUGH, Thomas A. (2017): Hippocrates' oath and Asclepius' snake. The birth of the medical profession. New York.

CHANIOTIS, Angelos (1995): Illness and Cures in the Greek Propitiatory Inscriptions and Dedications of Lydia and Phrygia. In: VAN DER EIJK/HORSTMANSHOFF/ SCHRIJVERS (1995), p. 323–334.

CHARITONIDOU, Angeliki (1978): Epidauros. Das Asklepios-Heiligtum und das Museum. Athen.

CHRIST, Karl (1995): Geschichte der Römischen Kaiserzeit. Von Augustus bis zu Konstantin. 3. Auflage. München.

CILLIERS, Louise; RETIEF, François P. (2013): Dream healing in Asclepieia in the Mediterranean. In: OBERHELMAN (2013), p. 69–92.

CLAUSS, Manfred (ed.) (1997a): Die römischen Kaiser. 55 historische Portraits von Caesar bis Iustinian. München.

CLAUSS, Manfred (1997b): Konstantin I. In: DERS. (1997a), p. 282–301.

CLAUSS, Manfred (1999): Kaiser und Gott. Herscherkult im Römischen Reich. Stuttgart, Leipzig.

CLINTON, Kevin (1994): The Epidauria and the Arrival of Asclepius in Athen. In: Hägg, Robin (ed.): Ancient Greek Cult Practice from the Epigraphical Evidence. Stockholm, p. 17–34.

COARELLI, Filippo (ed.) (1986): Fregellae 2. Il santuario di Esculapio. Roma.

COHN-HAFT, Louis (1956): The Public Physicians of Ancient Greece (= Smith College Studies in History, 42). Northampton (Mass.).

COMELLA, Annamaria (1981): Tipologia e diffusione dei complessi votivi in Italia in epoca medio- e tardo-repubblicana. In: Mélanges de l'École française de Rome. Moyen âge et temps modernes 93, p. 717–810.

COMELLA, Annamaria (1986): Il culto de Esculapio in Italia centrale durante il periodo reppublicane. In: COARELLI (1986), p. 145–152.

CORDES, Peter (1991): Innere Medizin bei Homer. In: Rheinisches Museum 134, p. 112–120.

CORDES, Peter (1994): Iatros. Das Bild des Arztes in der griechischen Literatur von Homer bis Aristoteles (= Palingenesia, 39). Stuttgart.

CROON, Johan H. (1986): Heilgötter. In: Reallexikon für Antike und Christentum 13, col. 1190–1232.

D

DEGRASSI, Donatella (1987): Interventi edilizi sull'isola Tiberina mel I sev. A. C.: Nota sulle testimonianze letterarie, epigrafiche ed archeologiche. In: Athenaeum 65, p. 521–527.

DEICHGRÄBER, Karl (1948): Die griechische Empirikerschule. Sammlung der Fragmente und Darstellung der Lehre. 2. Auflage. Berlin, Zürich.

DEICHGRÄBER, Karl (1950): Professio medici. Zum Vorwort des Scribonius Largus (= Abhandlungen der geistes- und sozialwissenschaftlichen Klasse, 9). Mainz.

DE FILIPPIS CAPPAI, Chiara (1991): Il culto di Asclepio da Epidauro a Roma: medicina del tempio e medicina scientifica. In: Civiltà classice e cristiana 12, p. 271–284.

DE LUCA, Gioia (1991): Zur Hygieia von Pergamon: ein Beitrag. In: Mitteilungen des Deutschen Archäologischen Instituts (Abteilung Istanbul) 41, p. 325–362.

DILLON, M. P. J. (1994): The Didactic Nature of the Epidaurian Iamata. In: Zeitschrift für Papyrologie und Epigraphik 101, p. 239–260.

DINGES, Martin (ed.) (2002a): Patients in the History of Homeopathy. Sheffield.

DINGES, Martin (2002b): Introduction: Patients in the History of Homeopathy. In: DINGES (2002a), p. 1–32.

DODDS, Eric R. (1970): Die Griechen und das Irrationale. Darmstadt.

DOW, Sterling; UPSON, Frieda p. (1944): The Foot of Sarapis. In: Hesperia 13, p. 58–77.

DÖRNEMANN, Michael (2013): Einer ist Arzt, Christus. Medizinales Verständnis von Erlösung in der Theologie der griechischen Kirchenväter des zweiten bis vierten Jahrhunderts. In: Zeitschrift für antikes Christentum 17, p. 102–124.

DRÄGER, Michael (1993): Die Städte der Provinz Asia in der Flavierzeit. Frankfurt/M.

DRAYCOTT, Jane; GRAHAM, Emma-Jayne (ed.) (2017): Bodies of Evidence. Ancient anatomical votives. Past, present and future (= Medicine and the body in antiquity). London.

DREXHAGE, Hans-Joachim (1981): Wirtschaft und Handel in den frühchristlichen Gemeinden (1.–3. Jh. n. Chr.). In: Römische Quartalsschrift für christliche Altertumskunde und für Kirchengeschichte 76, p. 1–72.

E

ECK, Werner (1997): Lateinische Epigraphik. In: GRAF, Fritz (ed.): Einleitung in die lateinische Philologie. Stuttgart, Leipzig, p. 92–111.

ECKART, Wolfgang U. (2013): Geschichte, Theorie und Ethik der Medizin. 7. Auflage. Berlin, Heidelberg, New York.

ECKART, Wolfgang U.; JÜTTE, Robert (2014): Medizingeschichte. Eine Einführung. 2. Auflage. Köln.

ERLER, Michael (ed.) (2000): Epikureismus in der späten Republik und der Kaiserzeit (= Philosophie der Antike, 11). Stuttgart.

ERNST, Katharina (1998): Patientengeschichte. Die kulturhistorische Wende in der Medizinhistoriographie. In: Bröer, Ralf (ed.): Eine Wissenschaft emanzipiert sich. Die

Medizinhistoriographie von der Aufklärung bis zur Postmoderne. Pfaffenweiler, p. 97–108.

F

FARNELL, Lewis R. (1921): Greek Hero Cults and Ideas of Immortality. Oxford.

FICHTNER, Gerhard (2018): Corpus Galenicum. Bibliographie der galenischen und pseudogalenischen Schriften. Berlin. Online: http://galen.bbaw.de/online-publications/Galen-Bibliographie_2018-06.pdf (6.7.2018).

FICHTNER, Gerhard (2017): Corpus Hippocraticum. Bibliographie der hippokratischen und pseudohippokratischen Werke. Berlin. Online: http://galen.bbaw.de/online-publications/Hippokrates-Bibliographie_2017-12.pdf (6.7.2018).

FISCHER, Klaus-Dietrich (1979): Kritisches zu den „Urkunden zur Hochschulpolitik der römischen Kaiser". In: Medizinhistorisches Journal 14, 312–321.

FORSÉN, Björn (1996): Griechische Gliederweihungen. Eine Untersuchung zu ihrer Typologie und ihrer religions- und sozialgeschichtlichen Bedeutung (= Papers and monographs of the Finnish institute at Athens, 4). Helsinki.

FRANKE, Peter R. (1969): Asklepios – Aesculapius auf antiken Münzen. In: Medizinischer Monatsspiegel 3, p. 60–67.

FRASER, Peter M. (1969): The Career of Erasistratus of Ceos. In: Rendiconti dell'Istituto Lombardo 103, p. 518–537.

FRON, Christian (2014): Der Reiz des Nil. Die Reise des Aelius Aristides nach Ägypten und ihr Einfluss auf seine Reden und Werke. In: OLSHAUSEN, Eckart; SAUER, Vera (ed.): Mobilität in den Kulturen der antiken Mittelmeerwelt (= Stuttgarter Kolloquium zur Historischen Geographie des Altertums, 11). Stuttgart, p. 205–224.

G

GARLAND, Robert (1992): Introducing New Gods. The politics of Athenian Religion. London.

GEERTZ, Clifford (1999): Dichte Beschreibung. Beiträge zum Verstehen kultureller Systeme. Frankfurt/M. [zuerst: Thick Description: Toward an interpretive theory of culture. In: GEERTZ, Clifford (ed.): The Interpretation of Cultures. Selected essays. 6. Auflage. New York 1973, p. 3–30].

GILLIAM, James F. (1961): The Plague under Marcus Aurelius. In: American Journal of Philology 82, p. 225–261.

GINOUVÈS, René (1962): Balaneutiké. Recherches sur le bain dans l'antiquité grecque. Paris.

GOLDER, Werner (2007): Hippokrates und das Corpus Hippocraticum. Eine Einführung für Philologen und Mediziner. Würzburg.

GONZÁLEZ SOUTELO, Silvia (2014): Medicine and Spas in the Roman Period. The Role of Doctors in Establishments with Mineral-Medicinal Waters. In: MICHAELIDES, Demetres (ed.): Medicine and healing in the ancient Mediterranean world. Oxford, p. 206–216.

GOULD, John (1973): Hiketeia. In: Journal of Hellenic Studies 93, p. 74–103.

GOUREVITCH, Danielle (1996): Wege der Erkenntnis: Medizin in der römischen Welt. In: GRMEK (1996), p. 114–150.

GUARDASOLE, Alessia (2005): Empiriker. In: LEVEN (2005), col. 254–255.

GRAF, Fritz (1992a): An Oracle against Pestilence from a Western Anatolian Town. In: Zeitschrift für Papyrologie und Epigraphik 92, p. 267–278.

GRAF, Fritz (1992b): Heiligtum und Ritual. Das Beispiel der griechisch-römischen Asklepieia. In: Schachter, Albert (ed.): Le sanctuaire grec (= Entretiens sur l'antiquité classique, 37). Genf, p. 157–199.

GRAF, Fritz (1996): Gottesnähe und Schadenszauber. Die Magie in der griechisch-römischen Antike. München.

GRAF, Fritz (1997): Asklepios I. Religion. In: Der Neue Pauly 1, col. 94–99.

GRAF, Fritz (1998): Heilgötter, Heilkult. IV. Griechenland und Rom. In: Der Neue Pauly 5, col. 243–247.

GRAUMANN, Lutz A. (2000): Die Krankengeschichten der Epidemienbücher des Corpus Hippocraticum. Medizinhistorische Bedeutung und Möglichkeiten der retrospektiven Diagnose. Aachen.

GRMEK, Mirko D.; GOUREVITCH, Danielle (1988): L'école médicale de Quintus et de Numisianus. In: Memoires du Centre Jean Parlerne 8, p. 43–60.

GRMEK, Mirko D. (1989): Diseases in the Ancient Greek World. Translated by Mireille Muellner and Leonard Muellner. Baltimore, London.

GRMEK, Mirko D. (ed.) (1996): Die Geschichte des medizinischen Denkens. Antike und Mittelalter. München.

GRMEK, Mirko D. (2000): Arétée de Cappadoce. Des causes et des signes des maladies aiguës et chroniques. Texte trad. par René T. H. Laënnec. Éd. par Mirko D. Grmek. Préf. de Danielle Gourevitch. Coll. Hautes études anciennes. Ecole Pratiques des Hautes Etudes Genève.

GRUEN, Erich p. (1993): Culture and National Identity in Republican Rome. London.

GRÜSSINGER, Ralf (ed.) (2011): Pergamon. Panorama der antiken Metropole. Begleitbuch zur Ausstellung. Eine Ausstellung der Antikensammlung der Staatlichen Museen zu Berlin. Petersberg.

GUARDUCCI, Margherita (1934): I „miracoli" di Asclepio a Labena. In: Historia 8, p. 410–428.

GÜNTHER, Linda-Marie (2000): Reisende und Pilger in der nordafrikanischen Hagiographie. In: Khanoussi, Moustapha; Ruggeri, Paola; Vismara, Cinzia (ed.): L'Africa Romana XIII. Atti del XIII convegno di studio, Djerba 1998. Rom, p. 413–417.

GUETTEL COLE, Susan (1988): The Uses of Water in Greek Sanctuaries. In: HÄGG, Robin; MARINATOS, Nanno; NORDQUIST, Gullög C. (ed.): Early Greek Cult Practice. Proceedings of the fifth international symposium at the Swedish institute at Athens. Stockholm, Göteborg, p. 161–165.

GUMMERUS, Herman (1932): Der Ärztestand im römischen Reich nach den Inschriften (= Societas Scientiarum Fennica. Commentationes Humanorum Litterarum, III 6). Helsingfors.

H

HABERLING, Wilhelm (1910): Die altrömischen Militärärzte. Berlin.

HABICHT, Christian (1959/60): Zwei neue Inschriften aus Pergamon. In: Istanbuler Mitteilungen 9/10, p. 109–127.

HAEHLING VON LANZENAUER, Brigitte (1996): Imperator soter. Der römische Kaiser als

Heilsbringer vor dem Hintergrund des Ringens zwischen Asklepioskult und Christusglaube. (= Düsseldorfer Arbeiten zur Geschichte der Medizin, 68). Düsseldorf.

HAFNER, German (1990): Die Ankunft des Asklepios-Schiffes in Ostia (292 v. u. Z.). In: Staatliche Museen zu Berlin (ed.): Forschungen und Berichte 28, p. 65–70.

HAHN, Johannes (1991): Plinius und die griechischen Ärzte in Rom. Naturkonzeption und Medizinkritik in der Naturalis Historia. In: Sudhoffs Archiv 75, p. 209–239.

HAHN, Peter Th. (1976): Die Weihinschrift des Apellas. Kurbericht oder Wundererzählung? Diss. med. Erlangen.

HALFMANN, Helmut (1979): Senatoren aus dem östlichen Teil des Imperium Romanum bis zum Ende des zweiten Jahrhunderts nach Christus. Göttingen.

HALFMANN, Helmut (2001): Städtebau und Bauherren im römischen Kleinasien. Ein Vergleich zwischen Pergamon und Ephesos (= Istanbuler Mitteilungen Beiheft, 43). Tübingen.

HAMILTON, Mary (1906): Incubation, or the Cure of Disease in Pagan Temples and Christian Churches. London.

HANSON, Ann E. (1997): Fragmentation and the Greek Medical Writers. In: Most, Glenn W. (ed.): Collecting fragments – Fragmente sammeln (= Aporemata, 1). Göttingen, p. 289–314.

HARIG, Georg (1971): Zum Problem „Krankenhaus" in der Antike. In: Klio 53, p. 179–195.

HARIG, Georg (1974): Bestimmungen der Intensität im medizinischen System Galens (= Schriften zur Geschichte und Kultur der Antike, 11). Berlin.

HARRIS, William V.; HOLMES, Brooke (ed.) (2008): Aelius Aristides between Greece, Rome and the Gods. Leiden, Boston.

HARRIS, William V. (ed.) (2016): Popular medicine in Graeco-Roman antiquity: Explorations (= Columbia Studies in the Classical Tradition, 42). Leiden, Boston.

HARRISSON, Juliette (2013): Dreams and dreaming in the Roman Empire. Cultural memory and imagination. London.

HARRISSON, Juliette (2014): The Development of the Practice of Incubation in the Ancient World. In: MICHAELIDES, Demetres (ed.): Medicine and healing in the ancient Mediterranean world. Oxford, p. 284–290.

HART, Gerald D. (2000): Asklepius the God of Medicine. Dorset.

HAUSMANN, Ulrich (1948): Kunst und Heiltum. Untersuchungen zu den griechischen Asklepiosreliefs. Potsdam.

HAUSSPERGER, Martha (2012): Die mesopotamische Medizin aus ärztlicher Sicht. Baden-Baden.

HAYMANN, Florian (2010): Caracalla in Aigeai: ein neues Tetradrachmon und weitere numismatische Belege. In: Jahrbuch für Numismatik und Geldgeschichte 60, p. 145–165.

HEIDERICH, Günter (1966): Asklepios. Gießen.

HEINZ, Werner (1996): Antike Balneologie in späthellenistischer und römischer Zeit. Zur medizinischen Wirkung römischer Bäder. In: ANRW II 37,3. Berlin, New York, p. 2411–2432.

HELCK, Wolfgang (1995): Die Beziehungen Ägyptens und Vorderasiens zur Ägäis bis ins 7. Jahrhundert v. Chr. (= Erträge der Forschung, 120). 2. Auflage. Darmstadt.

HENNING, Dirk (1989): Epidauros. In: Lauffer, Siegfried (ed.): Griechenland. Lexikon der historischen Stätten. Von den Anfängen bis zur Gegenwart. München, p. 219–221.

HERRMANN, Hans-Volkmar (1959): Omphalos. Münster.

HERZ, Peter (1997): Lokale Festkultur im Osten. In: CANCIK, Hubert; RÜPKE, Jörg (ed.): Römische Reichsreligion und Provinzialreligion. Tübingen, p. 239–264.

HERZOG, Rudolf (1899): Koische Forschungen und Funde. Leipzig. Reprint Hildesheim.

HERZOG, Rudolf (1931): Die Wunderheilungen von Epidauros. Ein Beitrag zur Geschichte der Medizin und der Religion (= Philologus Supplement, XXII 3). Leipzig.

HILLERT, Andreas (1990): Antike Ärztedarstellungen (= Marburger Schriften zur Medizingeschichte, 25). Frankfurt/M.

HOFFMANN, Michaela (1999): Griechische Bäder (= Quellen und Forschungen zur antiken Welt, 32). München.

HOHEISEL, Karl (1995): Religiöse und profane Formen nichtmedizinischen Heilens. In: DERS.; KLIMKEIT, Hans-Joachim (ed.): Heil und Heilung in den Religionen. Wiesbaden, p. 167–184.

HOLOWCHAK, M. Andrew (2001): Interpreting Dreams for Corrective Regimen: Diagnostic Dreams in Greco-Roman Medicine. In: Journal of the History of Medicine and Allied Sciences 56, p. 382–399.

HOLTZMANN, Bernard (1984): Asklepios. In: Lexicon Iconographicum Mythologiae Classicae II 1, p. 863–897.

HORSTMANSHOFF, H. F. J. (1992): Epidemie und Anomie in der griechischen Welt. In: Medizinhistorisches Journal 27, p. 43–65.

HULSKAMP, Maithe A. A. (2013): The value of dream diagnosis in the medical praxis of the Hippocratics and Galen. In: OBERHELMAN (2013), P. 33–68.

HUPFLOHER, Annette (2000): Kulte im kaiserzeitlichen Sparta: eine Rekonstruktion anhand der Priesterämter. Berlin.

I

IAKOVIDIS, Spyros E. (1985): Mykene – Epidauros – Argos – Tiryns – Nauplia. Vollständiger Führer durch die Museen und archäologischen Stätten der Argolis. Athen.

INTERDONATO, Elisabetta (2013): L' Asklepieion di Kos. Archeologia del culto (= Supplementi e monografie della rivista "Archeologia classica", 12 = N. S. 9). Roma.

ISRAELOWICH, Ido (2012): Society, medicine and religion in the sacred tales of Aelius Aristides. Leiden.

ISRAELOWICH, Ido (2015): Patients and healers in the High Roman Empire. Baltimore.

ISRAELOWICH, Ido (2016): Medical care in the Roman army during the High Empire. In: HARRIS (2016), p. 215–230.

J

JACKSON, Ralph (1988): Doctors and Diseases in the Roman Empire. London.

JACOBOVITS, Immanuel (1959): Jewish Medical Ethics. A comparative and historical study of the Jewish religious attitude to medicine and its practice. New York.

JANKRIFT, Kay Peter (ed.) (2003): Krankheit und Heilkunde im Mittelalter. Darmstadt.

JAYNE, Walter A. (1925): The Healing Gods of Ancient Civilizations. New York.

JONES, Arnold H. M. (1971): The Cities of the Eastern Roman Provinces. 2. Auflage. Oxford.

JONES, Christopher P. (2012): Galen's Travels. In: Chiron 42, p. 399–419.

JOST, Madeleine (1985): Sanctuaires et cultes d'Arcadie. Paris.

JOUANNA, Jacques (1996): Die Entstehung der Heilkunst im Westen. In: GRMEK (1996), p. 28–80.

JÜTTE, Robert (1990): Sozialgeschichte der Medizin: Inhalte – Methoden – Ziele. In: Medizin, Gesellschaft und Geschichte 9, p. 149–164.

JÜTTE, Robert (1991): Ärzte, Heiler und Patienten. Medizinischer Alltag in der frühen Neuzeit. München, Zürich.

JÜTTE, Robert (1994): Bader, Barbiere und Hebammen. Heilkundige als Randgruppen? In: HERGEMÖLLER, Bernd-Ulrich (ed.): Randgruppen der spätmittelalterlichen Gesellschaft. Ein Hand- und Studienbuch. 2. Auflage. Warendorf, p. 89–120.

JÜTTE, Robert (1996): Samuel Hahnemanns Patientenschaft. In: DINGES, Martin (ed.): Homöopathie. Patienten – Heilkundige – Institutionen. Von den Anfängen bis heute. Heidelberg, p. 23–44.

K

KÁKOSY, László (1989): Zauberei im alten Ägypten. Leipzig.

KAMPMANN, Ursula (1992/3): Asklepios mit Omphalos in der römischen Reichsprägung. Zu einem Beispiel der Beeinflussung der Reichsprägung durch Lokalmünzen. In: Jahrbuch für Numismatik und Geldgeschichte 42/43, p. 39–48.

KARENBERG, Axel; LEITZ, Christian (ed.) (2000): Heilkunde und Hochkultur I. Geburt, Seuche und Traumdeutung in den antiken Zivilisationen des Mittelmeerraumes (= Naturwissenschaft – Philosophie – Geschichte, 14). Münster.

KATAKES, Stylianos E. (2002): Epidauros. Ta glypta tōn Rōmaïkōn chronōn apo to Iero tu Apollōnos Maleata kai tu Asklēpiu. Vol. 2. Athen.

KAVVADIAS, Panagiotes (1883): Ἐπιγραφαὶ. Ἐκ τῶν ἐν Ἐπιδαυρίᾳ ἀνασκαφῶν. In: Archailogikè Ephèmeris 22, p. 197–238.

KAVVADIAS, Panagiotes (1885): Ἐπιγραφαὶ. Ἐκ τῶν ἐν Ἐπιδαυρίᾳ ἀνασκαφῶν. In: Archailogikè Ephèmeris 24, p. 65–86.

KAVVADIAS, Panagiotes (1893): Fouilles d' Épidaure. Athen.

KAVVADIAS, Panagiotes (1900): Τὸ ἱερὸν τοῦ Ἀσκληπιοῦ ἐν Ἐπιδαύρῳ καὶ ἡ θεραπεία τῶν ἀσθενῶν. Athen.

KERÉNYI, Karl (1956): Der göttliche Arzt. Studien über Asklepios und seine Kultstätten. Darmstadt.

KING, Daniel (2017): Experiencing pain in Imperial Greek culture. Oxford.

KISLINGER, Ewald (2005): Ärztin. In: LEVEN (2005), col. 16–17.

KLOSS, Gerrit (2001): Sokrates, ein Hahn für Asklepios und die Pflege der Seelen. Ein neuer Blick auf den Schluß von Platons Phaidon. In: Gymnasium 108, p. 223–240.

KNIBBE, Dieter (1981): Quandocumque quis trium virorum rei publicae constituendae. Ein neuer Fund aus Ephesos. In: Zeitschrift für Papyrologie und Epigraphik 44, p. 1–10.

KNIBBE, Dieter (1982): Neue Inschriften aus Ephesos VIII. In: Jahreshefte des Österreichischen Archäologischen Instituts 53, p. 136–140.

KOELBING, Huldrych M. (1977): Arzt und Patient in der antiken Welt. Zürich, München.

KOETTING, Bernhard (1980): Peregrinatio religiosa. Wallfahrten in der Antike und das Pilgerwesen in der alten Kirche. 2. Auflage. Münster.

KOLLESCH, Jutta (1965): Galen und seine ärztlichen Kollegen. In: Altertum 11, p. 47–53.

KOLLESCH, Jutta (1979): Ärztliche Ausbildung in der Antike. In: Klio 61, p. 507–513.

KOLLESCH, Jutta (1981): Galen und die Zweite Sophistik. In: NUTTON (1981), p. 1–11.

KOLLESCH, Jutta; NICKEL, Diethard (1994): Bibliographia Galeniana. Die Beiträge des 20. Jahrhunderts zur Galenforschung. In: ANRW II 37,2. Berlin, New York, p. 1351–1420.

KOLTA, Kamal S.; SCHWARZMANN-SCHAFHAUSER, Doris (2000): Die Heilkunde im alten Ägypten. Magie und Ratio in der Krankheitsvorstellung und therapeutischen Praxis (= Sudhoffs Archiv Beiheft, 42). Stuttgart.

KORENJAK, Martin (2005): „Unbelievable confusion". Weshalb sind die „Hieroi Logoi" des Aelius Aristides so wirr? In: Hermes 133, p. 215–234.

KORPELA, Jukka (1987): Das Medizinalpersonal im antiken Rom. Eine sozialgeschichtliche Untersuchung (= Annales academiae scientiarum fennicae. Dissertationes humanarum litterarum, 45). Helsinki.

KOTANSKY, Roy (1991): Incantations and Prayers for Salvation in Inscribed Greek Amulets. In: FARAONE, Christopher A.; OBBINK, Dirk (ed.): Magica Hiera. Ancient Greek magic and religion. New York, Oxford, p. 107–137.

KÖRNER, Otto (1929): Die ärztlichen Kenntnisse in Ilias und Odyssee. München.

KRANZ, Peter (1990): Zeugnisse hadrianischer Religionspolitik im Osten. In: BÖRKER, Christoph; DONDERER, Michael (ed.): Das antike Rom und der Osten. Festschrift Klaus Perlasca. Erlangen, p. 125–141.

KRANZ, Peter (2004): Pergameus Deus. Archäologische und numismatische Studien zu den Darstellungen des Asklepios in Pergamon während Hellenismus und Kaiserzeit. Mit einem Exkurs zur Überlieferung statuarischer Bildwerke in der Antike. Möhnesee.

KRANZ, Peter (2010): Hygieia. Die Frau an Asklepios' Seite. Untersuchungen zu Darstellung und Funktion in klassischer und hellenistischer Zeit unter Einbeziehung der Gestalt des Asklepios. Möhnesee.

KRAUSS, Friedrich (1944): Die Prora an der Tiberinsel in Rom. In: Mitteilungen des Deutschen Archäologischen Instituts, Römische Abteilung 59, p. 159–172.

KRUG, Antje (1993): Heilkunst und Heilkult. Medizin in der Antike. 2. Auflage. München.

KUDLIEN, Fridolf (1967): Der Beginn des medizinischen Denkens bei den Griechen. Von Homer bis Hippokrates. Zürich.

KUDLIEN, Fridolf (1978): Beichte und Heilung. In: Medizinhistorisches Journal 13, p. 1–14.

KUDLIEN, Fridolf (1985): Jüdische Ärzte im Römischen Reich. In: Medizinhistorisches Journal 20, p. 36–57.

KUDLIEN, Fridolf (1986): Die Stellung des Arztes in der römischen Gesellschaft. Freigeborene, Römer, Eingebürgerte, Peregrine, Sklaven, Freigelassene als Ärzte (= Forschungen zur antiken Sklaverei, 18). Stuttgart.

KUDLIEN, Fridolf (1988): Heiltätige Scharlatane und Quacksalber in der Antike – eine

Randgruppe der Gesellschaft? In: Weiler, Ingomar (ed.): Soziale Randgruppen und Außenseiter im Altertum. Graz, p. 137–168.

KUDLIEN, Fridolf; DURLING, Richard J. (ed.) (1991): Galen's Method of Healing. Leiden.

KULLMANN, Wolfgang; ALTHOFF, Jochen; ASPER, Markus (ed.) (1998): Gattungen wissenschaftlicher Literatur in der Antike (= ScriptOralia, 95). Tübingen.

KÜNZL, Ernst (1991): Die medizinische Versorgung der römischen Armee zur Zeit des Kaiser Augustus und die Reaktion der Römer auf die Situation bei den Kelten und Germanien. In: Aßkamp, Rudolf (ed.): Die römische Okkupation nördlich der Alpen zur Zeit des Augustus. Kolloquium Berkamen 1989. Vorträge (= Bodenaltertümer Westfalens, 26). Münster, p. 185–202.

KYRIELEIS, Helmut (1979): Babylonische Bronzen im Heraion von Samos. In: Jahrbuch des Deutschen Archäologischen Instituts 94, p. 32–48.

L

LABISCH, Alfons (2005a): Dogmatiker. In: LEVEN (2005), col. 233–234.

LABISCH, Alfons (2005b): Methodiker. In: LEVEN (2005), col. 613–614.

LACHMUND, Jens; STOLLBERG, Gunnar (ed.) (1992): The Social Construction of Illness. Illness and medical knowledge in past and present (= Medizin, Gesellschaft und Geschichte Beiheft, 1). Stuttgart.

ŁAJTAR, Adam (2006): Deir el-Bahari in the Hellenistic and Roman Periods. A study of an Egyptian temple based on Greek sources (= The journal of juristic papyrology, Supplement, 4). Warszawa.

LANG, Mabel L. (1977): Cure and Cult in Ancient Corinth. A guide to the Asklepieion. Princeton.

LANGHOLF, Volker (1996): Lukian und die Medizin: Zu einer tragischen Katharsis bei den Abderiten (De historia conscribenda § 1). In: ANRW II 37,3, p. 2793–2841.

LE GLAY, Marcel (1978): Hadrien et l'Asklépieion de Pergame. In: Bulletin de correspondance hellénique 100, p. 347–372.

LECOS, E. P.; PENTOGALOS, Gerasimos E. (ed.) (1986): Early and Late Asclepieia. Similarities and differences. In: Ancient and popular healing. Symposium on ancient medicine, Athens 4–10 Oktober 1986. Finnish Institutes Athens. Vammala, p. 13–24.

LEITH, David (2016): How popular were the medical sects? In: HARRIS (2016), p. 231–250.

LEVEN, Karl-Heinz (1987): Medizinisches bei Eusebios von Kaisareia (= Düsseldorfer Arbeiten zur Geschichte der Medizin, 62). Düsseldorf.

LEVEN, Karl-Heinz (1991): Thukydides und die „Pest" in Athen. In: Medizinhistorisches Journal 26, p. 128–160.

LEVEN, Karl-Heinz (1997a): Die Geschichte der Infektionskrankheiten. Von der Antike bis ins 20. Jahrhundert. Landsberg/L.

LEVEN, Karl-Heinz (1997b): Asklepios. Inschriften, Wunderberichte. Seit dem 4. Jh. v. Chr. In: SCHÜTZE, Oliver (ed.): Metzler Lexikon antiker Autoren. Stuttgart, Weimar, p. 115–116.

LEVEN, Karl-Heinz (1998): Krankheiten – historische Deutung versus retrospektive Diagnose. In: PAUL/SCHLICH (1998), p. 153–185.

LEVEN, Karl-Heinz (2004): „At times these ancient facts seem to lie before me like a patient on a hospital bed" – Retrospektive Diagnosis and Ancient Medical History.

In: HORSTMANSHOFF, Herman F. J.; STOL, Marten (ed.): Magic and Rationality in Ancient Near Eastern and Graeco-Roman Medicine. Leiden, p. 369–386.

LEVEN, Karl-Heinz (ed.) (2005): Antike Medizin. Ein Lexikon. München.

LEVICK, Barbara (1999): Vespasian. London.

LEY, Anne (1997): Asklepios II. Ikonographie. In: Der Neue Pauly 1, p. 99–100.

LIDONNICI, Lynn R. (1992): Compositional Background of the Epidaurian ἰάματα: In: American Journal of Philology 113, p. 25–41.

LINDGREN, Uta (1978): Frühformen abendländischer Hospitäler im Lichte einiger Bedingungen ihrer Entstehung. In: Historia Hospitalium 12 (1977/78), p. 32–61.

LLOYD, Geoffrey E. R. (1979): Magic, Reason and Experience. Studies in the origin and development of Greek science. Cambridge.

LO CASCIO, Elio (ed.) (2012): L' impatto della „peste antonina". Quinto degli Incontri Capresi di Storia dell'Econimia Antica. Roma e Anacapri nei giorni 8–11 ottobre 2008 (= Pragmateiai, 22). Bari.

LORENZ, Günther (1988): Apollon, Asklepios und Hygieia. Drei Typen von Heilgöttern aus der Sicht der vergleichenden Religionsgeschichte. In: Saeculum 39, p. 1–11.

LORENZ, Günther (2000): Tiere im Leben der alten Kulturen. Schriftlose Kulturen, Alter Orient, Ägypten, Griechenland und Rom (= Alltag und Kultur im Altertum, 5). Wien, Köln, Weimar.

LORENZ, Günther (2004): Asklepios, der Heiler mit dem Hund und der Orient. In: ULF, Christoph; ROLLINGER, Robert (ed.): Griechische Archaik. Interne Entwicklungen – Externe Impulse. Berlin, p. 335–365.

LORENZ, Günther (2016): Asklepios, der Heiler mit dem Hund, und der Orient. Religion und Medizin in alten Kulturen in universalhistorischer Sicht. Innsbruck.

M

MALITZ, Jürgen (1997): Vespasian. In: CLAUSS (1997a), p. 86–94.

MANLEY, Jennifer (2014): Measles and ancient plagues. A note on new scientific evidence. In: Classical World 107, p. 393–397.

MANN, CHRISTIAN (2011): „Um keinen Kranz, um das Leben kämpfen wir!" Gladiatoren im Osten des Römischen Reiches und die Frage der Romanisierung. Berlin.

MÄNNLEIN-ROBERT, Irmgard (2015): Iamatika. In: SEIDENSTICKER, Bernd; STÄHLI, Adrian; WESSELS, Antje (ed.): Der Neue Poseidipp. Text – Übersetzung – Kommentar. Darmstadt, p. 343–374.

MARASCO, Gabriele (1995): L'introduction de la médecine grecque à Rome: une dissension politique et idéologique. In: VAN DER EIJK/HORSTMANSHOFF/SCHRIJVERS (1995), p. 35–48.

MARKSCHIES, Christoph (2006): Gesund werden im Schlaf? Die antiken Schlafkulte und das Christentum. In: Theologische Literaturzeitung 131, p. 1233–1244.

MARTIN, Roland; METZGER, Henri (1976): La religion grecque. Paris.

MARTZAVOU, Paraskevi (2012): Dream, Narrative, and the construction of hope in the 'Healing Miracles' of Epidauros. In: Angelos Chaniotis (ed.): Sources and methods for the study of emotions in the Greek world (= Heidelberger althistorische Beiträge und epigraphische Studien, 52), Stuttgart, p. 177–204.

MATTERN, Susan P. (2013): The Prince of Medicine. Galen in the Roman Empire. Oxford.

MATTINGLY, Harold; CARSON, Robert A. G.; HILL, Philip V. (1975): Coins of the Roman Empire in the British Museum. Pertinax to Elagabalus. 2. Auflage. London.

MAUL, Stefan M. (2001): Die Heilkunde im Alten Orient. In: Medizinhistorisches Journal 36, p. 3–22.

MCCASLAND, p. Vernon (1939): The Asclepios Cult in Palestine. In: Journal of Biblical Literature 58, p. 221–227.

MEDICK, Hans (2001): Quo vadis Historische Anthropologie? Geschichtsforschung zwischen Historischer Kulturwissenschaft und Mikro-Historie. In: Historische Anthropologie 9, p. 78–92.

MEIER, Carl A. (1967): Ancient Incubation and Modern Psychotherapy. Illinois.

MEIER, Mischa (1999): Beobachtungen zu den sogenannten Pestschilderungen bei Thukydides II 47–54 und bei Prokop, Bell. Pers. II 22–23. In: Tyche 14, p. 177–210.

MEISSNER, Burkhard (1997): Berufsausbildung in der Antike (Rom und Griechenland). In: Liedtke, Max (ed.): Berufliche Bildung – Geschichte, Gegenwart, Zukunft. Bad Heilbrunn, p. 55–99.

MEISSNER, Burkhard (1999): Die technologische Fachliteratur der Antike. Struktur, Überlieferung und Wirkung technischen Wissens in der Antike; (ca. 400 v. Chr.–ca. 500 n. Chr.). Berlin.

MELFI, Milena (2007): I Santuari di Asclepio in Grecia. Vol. 1. Rom.

MERKELBACH, Reinhold (2001): Isis Regina – Zeus Sarapis. Die griechisch-ägyptische Religion nach den Quellen dargestellt. 2. Auflage. Stuttgart.

MEYER, Marion (1988): Erfindung und Wirkung. Zum Asklepios Giustini. In: Mitteilungen des Deutschen Archäologischen Instituts (Abteilung Athen) 103, p. 119–159.

MEYER, Marion (1994): Zwei Asklepiostypen des 4. Jahrhunderts v. Chr.: Asklepios Giustini und Asklepios Athen-Macerata. In: BORBEIN, Adolf H. (ed.): Antike Plastik 23. Herausgegeben im Auftrag des Deutschen Archäologischen Instituts. München, p. 7–55.

MEYER-STEINEG, Theodor (1916): Das medizinische System der Methodiker. Eine Vorstudie zu Caelius Aurelianus „De morbis acutis et chronicis". Jena.

MEYER-ZWIFFELHOFFER, Eckhard (2002): Politikôs archein. Zum Regierungsstil der senatorischen Statthalter in den kaiserzeitlichen griechischen Provinzen. Stuttgart.

MIKALSON, Jon D. (1984). Religion and Plague in Athens, 431–423 B. C. In: RIGSBY, Kent J. (ed.): Studies presented to Sterling Dow on his eightieth birthday. Durham, p. 217–225.

MONTEVECCHI, Orsolina (1981): Vespasiano acclimato dagli Alessandri. Atti del Congresso Internazionale di Studi Vespasianei. Rieti, p. 483–495.

MORENZ, Siegfried (1949/50): Vespasian, Heiland der Kranken. Persönliche Frömmigkeit im antiken Herrscherkult? In: Würzburger Jahrbücher für die Altertumswissenschaft 4, p. 370–378.

MOST, Glenn W. (1993): A Cock for Asclepius. In: Classical Quarterly 43, p. 96–111.

MUDRY, Philippe (1989): Malade et dévot d'Asclépios: l'autobiographie d'Aelius Aristide. In: Revue medicales de la Suisse romande 109, p. 979–985.

MUDRY, Philippe (1994a): Le ‚De medicina‘ de Celse. Rapport bibiliographique. In: ANRW 37,1. Berlin, New York, p. 787–799.

MUDRY, Philippe (1994b): L'orientation doctrinale du ‚De medicina‘ de Cels. In: ANRW 37,1. Berlin, New York, p. 800–818.

MÜLLER, Helmut (1987): Ein Heilungsbericht aus dem Asklepieion von Pergamon. In: Chiron 17, p. 191–233.

MÜLLER, Helmut (2011): Pergamon als Polis. Institutionen, Ämter und Bevölkerung. In: GRÜSSINGER (2011), p. 254–259.

MYLONAS, Georgios E. (1961): Eleusis and the Eleusinian mysteries. Princeton.

N

NEUGEBAUER, Karl Anton (1921): Asklepios. Ein Beitrag zur Kritik römischer Statuenkopien. Berlin.

NUTTON, Vivian (1970): The Doctors of the Roman Navy. In: Epigraphica 32, p. 66–71.

NUTTON, Vivian (1972): Roman Oculists. In: Epigraphica 34, p. 16–29.

NUTTON, Vivian (1973): The Chronology of Galen's Early Career. In: Classical Quarterly 67, p. 158–171.

NUTTON, Vivian (ed.) (1981): Galen. Problems and Prospects. London.

NUTTON, Vivian (1995a): Galen ad multos annos. In: Dynamis 15, p. 25–40.

NUTTON, Vivian (1995b): The Medical Meeting Place. In: VAN DER EIJK/HORSTMANS-HOFF/ SCHRIJVERS (1995), p. 3–25.

NUTTON, Vivian (1997): Empiriker. In: Der Neue Pauly 3, col. 1016–1018.

NUTTON, Vivian (1999a): Krankenhaus. In: Der Neue Pauly 6, col. 789–793.

NUTTON, Vivian (1999b): Medizin. IV. Klassische Antike. In: Der Neue Pauly 7, col. 1107–1117.

NUTTON, Vivian (2004): Ancient medicine. London, New York.

O

OBERHELMAN, Steven M. (1993): Dreams in Graeco-roman Medicine. In: ANRW II 37,1. Berlin, New York, p. 121–156.

OBERHELMAN, Steven M. (1997): Aretaeus of Cappadocia: the Pneumatic physician of the first century A. D. In: ANRW II 37,2. Berlin, New York, p. 941–996.

OBERHELMAN, Steven M. (ed.) (2013): Dreams, Healing, and Medicine in Greece. From Antiquity to the Present. Farnham, Burlington.

OEHLER, Johann (1909): Epigraphische Beiträge zur Geschichte des Ärztestandes. In: Janus 14, p. 4–20 u. 111–123.

OHLEMUTZ, Erwin (1940): Die Kulte und Heiligtümer der Götter in Pergamon. Würzburg.

OSER-GROTE, Carolin (1998): Medizinische Schriftsteller. In: FLASHAR, Hellmut (ed.): Überweg. Grundriß der Geschichte der Philosophie. Die Philosophie der Antike. Vol. 2,1. Basel, p. 457–485.

P

PAPACHATZIS, Nikos (1978): Mykene – Epidauros – Tiryns – Nauplia. Führer durch die klassischen Stätten der Argolis. Athen.

PARKER, Robert (1983): Miasma. Pollution and purification in early Greek religion. Oxford.

PARKER, Robert (1997): Athenian Religion. A History. Oxford.

PAUL, Norbert; SCHLICH, Thomas (ed.) (1998): Medizingeschichte: Aufgaben, Probleme, Perspektiven. Frankfurt/M., New York.

PEARCY, Lee T. (1988): Theme, Dream and Narrative: Reading the sacred tales of Aelius Aristides. In: Transactions and Proceedings of the American Philological Association 118, p. 377–391.

PENN, Raymond G. (1994): Medicine on Ancient Greek and Roman Coins. London.

PENSABENE, Patrizio; RIZZO, Marino A.; ROGHI, Maria; TALAMO, Emilia (1980): Terracotte votive dal Tevere. Rom.

PERNOT, Laurent (2008): Aelius Aristides and Rome. In: HARRIS/HOLMES (2008), p. 175–201.

PETRIDOU, Georgia; THUMIGER, Chiara (ed.) (2016): Homo patiens. Approaches to the patient in the ancient world (= Studies in Ancient Medicine, 45). Leiden.

PETSALIS-DIOMIDIS, Alexia (2010): Truly beyond wonders. Aelius Aristides and the cult of Asklepios. Oxford, New York.

PETZOLDT, Leander (ed.) (1978). Magie und Religion. Beiträge zu einer Theorie der Magie (= Wege der Forschung, 337). Darmstadt.

PFEFFER, Marina E. (1969): Einrichtungen der sozialen Sicherung in der griechischen und römischen Antike unter besonderer Berücksichtigung der Sicherung bei Krankheit. Berlin.

PIGEAUD, Jackie (1982): Sur le méthodisme. In: SABBAH, Guy (ed.): Médecins et Médecine dans l'Antiquité. Actes des journées d'étude sur la médecine antique d'époque romaine. Mémoires III du Centre Jean Palerne. Saint-Étienne, p. 181–183.

POMEROY, Sarah B. (1997): Families in Classical and Hellenistic Greece. Representation and realities. Oxford.

PORTER, Roy (1985a): The Patient's View: Doing medical history from below. In: Theory and Society 14, p. 175–198.

PORTER, Roy (ed.) (1985b): Patients and Practitioners. Lay Perceptions of Medicine in Preindustrial Societies. Cambridge.

PORTER, Roy; PORTER, Dorothy (1988): In Sickness and Health. The British Experience 1650–1850. London.

PORTER, Roy (2000): Die Kunst des Heilens. Eine medizinische Geschichte der Menschheit von der Antike bis heute. Darmstadt.

PRATSCH, Thomas (2013): „... erwachte und war geheilt". Inkubationsdarstellungen in byzantinischen Heiligenviten. In: Zeitschrift für antikes Christentum 17, p. 68–86.

PRICE, Simon R. F. (1984): Rituals and Power. The Roman imperial cult in Asia minor. Cambridge.

PRICE, Simon R. F. (2004): The future of dreams. From Freud to Artemidorus. In: OSBORNE, Robin (ed.): Studies in ancient Greek and Roman society. Cambridge, p. 226–259.

PRIOR, Lindsay (1992): The Local Space of Medical Discourse. Disease, illness and hospital architecture. In: LACHMUND/STOLLBERG (1992), p. 67–84.

R

RADT, Wolfgang (1999): Pergamon. Geschichte und Bauten einer antiken Metropole. Darmstadt.

RECHENAUER, Georg (2000): Rez. zu CORDES (1994). In: Gnomon 5, p. 385–389.

RENBERG, Gil H. (2017): Where dreams may come. Incubation sanctuaries in the Greco-Roman World. 2 vols. (= Religions in the Graeco-Roman World, 184). Leiden.

RENGSTORFF, Karl H. (1953): Die Anfänge der Auseinandersetzung zwischen Christusglaube und Asklepiosfrömmigkeit (= Schriften der Gesellschaft zur Förderung der Westfälischen Landesuniversität zu Münster, 30). Münster.

RICHTER, Daniel S.; JOHNSON, William A. (ed.) (2017): The Oxford Handbook of the Second Sophistic. Oxford.

RIDDLE, John M. (1985): Dioscorides on Pharmacy and Medicine. Austin (Texas).

RIDDLE, John M. (1994): High Medicine and Low Medicine. In: ANRW 37,1. Berlin, New York, p. 102–120.

RIETHMÜLLER, Jürgen W. (1996): Die Tholos und das Ei – Zur Deutung der Thymele in Epidauros. In: Nikephoros 9, p. 71–109.

RIETHMÜLLER, Jürgen W. (2005): Asklepios. Heiligtümer und Kulte. 2 Vols. (= Studien zu antiken Heiligtümern, 2,1–2). Heidelberg.

RIETHMÜLLER, Jürgen W. (2011): Das Asklepieion von Pergamon. In: GRÜSSINGER (2011), p. 228–234.

RISSE, Guenter B. (1999): Mending Bodies, Saving Souls. A history of hospitals. New York, Oxford.

ROBERT, Fernand (1939): Thymele (= BEAR, 147). Paris.

ROBERT, Louis (1940): Les gladiateurs dans l'orient grec. Paris.

ROBERT, Louis (1973): De Cilicie à Messine et à Plymouth avec deux inscriptions grecques errantes. In: Journal des Savants, p. 162–211 (= Opera minora selecta, 7. Amsterdam 1990, p. 225–275).

ROBERT, Louis (1978): Monnaies et textes grecs. In: Journal des Savants, p. 145–163.

ROBERT, Louis (1980): À travers l'Asie Mineure. Athen.

ROELCKE, Volker (1998): Medikale Kultur: Möglichkeiten und Grenzen der Anwendung eines kulturwissenschaftlichen Konzepts in der Medizingeschichte. In: PAUL/ SCHLICH (1998), p. 45–68.

ROESCH, Paul (1982): Le culte d'Asclépios à Rome. In: Sabbah, Guy (ed.): Médecins et médecine dans l'antiquité (= Centre Jean Palerne Mém., 3). St. Etienne, p. 171–179.

ROSENTHAL, Franz (1956): In hippocratis Iusiurandum commentarii. In: Bulletin of the History of Medicine 30, p. 52–87.

RUSSELL, David A.; TRAPP, Michael; NESSELRATH, Heinz-Günther (2016) (ed.): Aelius Aristides. Selected Prose Hymns. Introduction, text, translation and interpretative essays (= Scripta ANtiquitatis Posterioris ad Ethicam Religionemque pertinentia, 29). Tübingen.

RÜTTIMANN, René J. (1986): Asclepius and Jesus. The form, character and status of the Asclepius cult in the second-century C.E. and its significance in early christianity. Diss. Harvard. University. Cambridge (Mass.).

S

SAMAMA, Évelyne (2003): Les médecins dans le monde grec. Sources épigraphiques sur la naissance d'un corps médical (= École Pratique de Hautes Études, Sciences Historiques et Philologiques 3, Hautes études du monde gréco-romain, 31). Genève.

SAMAMA, Évelyne (2017): La médecine de guerre en Grèce ancienne (= De diversis artibus, 98). Turnhout.

SCARBOROUGH, John (1969): Roman Medicine. London.

SCARBOROUGH, John (1971): Galen and the Gladiators. In: Episteme 5, p. 98–111.

SCHADEWALDT, Hans (1967): Asklepios und Christus. In: Medizinische Welt 31, p. 1755–1761.

SCHÄFER, Daniel (2000): Traum und Wunderheilung im Asklepios-Kult und in der griechisch-römischen Medizin. In: KARENBERG/LEITZ (2000), p. 259–274.

SCHEER, Tanja p. (1993): Mythische Vorväter. Zur Bedeutung griechischer Heroenmythen im Selbstverständnis kleinasiatischer Städte. München.

SCHEER, Tanja p. (2000): Die Gottheit und ihr Bild. Untersuchungen zur Funktion griechischer Kultbilder in Religion und Politik (= Zetemata, 105). München.

SCHLANGE-SCHÖNINGEN (2003), Heinrich: Die römische Gesellschaft bei Galen. Berlin, New York.

SCHLUMBOHM, Jürgen (ed.) (1998): Mikrogeschichte – Makrogeschichte, komplementär oder inkommensurabel. Göttingen.

SCHNALKE, Thomas (1990): Asklepios – Heilgott und Heilkult. In: Ders. (ed.): Asklepios – Heilgott und Heilkult. 12.7.–30.9.1990. Konzeption, Gestaltung und Texte Thomas Schnalke und Claudia Selheim. Erlangen.

SCHNALKE, Thomas (2005): Asklepios-Schlange. In: LEVEN (2005), col. 112–113.

SCHNALKE, Thomas; WITTERN, Renate (1993): Asklepios trifft Hippokrates. Zum Verhältnis von religiöser und wissenschaftlich-rationaler Medizin in der griechisch-römischen Antike. In: Jahrbuch des Deutschen Medizinhistorischen Museums 7 (1993), p. 85–103 (= also In: KEMPER, Peter (ed.): Die Geheimnisse der Gesundheit. Medizin zwischen Heilkunde und Heiltechnik. Frankfurt/M. 1994, p. 95–114).

SCHÖNER, Erich (1964): Das Viererschema in der antiken Humoralpathologie (= Sudhoffs Archiv Beiheft, 4). Wiesbaden.

SCHOUTEN, Jan (1967): The Rod and Serpent of Asklepios. Symbol of medicine. Amsterdam.

SCHRÖDER, Heinrich O. (1988): Publius Aelius Aristides. Ein kranker Rhetor im Ringen um den Sinn seines Lebens. In: Gymnasium 95, p. 375–380.

SCHUBERT, Charlotte (2005): Der hippokratische Eid. Medizin und Ethik von der Antike bis heute. Darmstadt.

SCHULZE, Christian (1999): Aulus Cornelius Celsus – Arzt oder Laie? Autor, Konzept, und Adressaten der „De medicina libri octo" (= BAC, 42). Trier.

SCHULZE, Christian (2005): Medizin und Christentum in Spätantike und frühem Mittelalter. Christliche Ärzte und ihr Wirken. Tübingen.

SCHULZE, Joachim-Friedrich (1971): Die Entwicklung der Medizin in Rom und das Verhältnis der Römer gegenüber der ärztlichen Tätigkeit von den Anfängen bis zum Beginn der Kaiserzeit. In: Živa Antika (Antiquité vivante) 21, p. 485–505.

SCHUMACHER, Joseph (1963): Antike Medizin. Die naturphilosophischen Grundlagen der Medizin in der griechischen Antike. 2. Auflage. Berlin.

SCHUMACHER, Leonhard (2001): Sklaverei in der Antike. Alltag und Schicksal der Unfreien. München.

SCHWINDEN, Lothar (1994): Die Weihinschrift für Asclepius CIL XII 3636 aus Trier. In: Trierer Zeitschrift für Geschichte und Kunst des Trierer Landes und seiner Trier Nachbargebiete 57, p. 133–145.

SCONOCCHIA, Sergio (1994): L'opera di Scribonio Largo e la letteratura medica latina del 1 sec. d. C. In: ANRW 37,1. Berlin, New York, p. 843–922.

SELINGER, Reinhard (1999): Experimente mit dem Skalpell am menschlichen Körper in der griechisch-römischen Antike. In: Saeculum 50, p. 29–47.

SHERWIN-WHITE, Susan M. (1978): Ancient Cos. An historical study from the Dorian settlement to the imperial period (= Hypomnemata, 51). Göttingen.

SIEBENTHAL, Wolf von (1950): Krankheit als Folge der Sünde (= Heilkunde und Geisteswelt. Eine medizinhistorische Schriftenreihe, 2). Hannover.

SIEFERT, Helmut (1980): Inkubation, Imagination und Kommunikation im antiken Asklepioskult. Katathymes Bildererleben. Wien.

SMARCZYK, Bernhard (1984): Untersuchungen zur Religionspolitik und politischen Propaganda Athens im Delisch-Attischen Seebund. München.

SMITH, Martin F. (1993): Diogenes of Oinoanda. The Epicurean Inscription. Neapel.

SMITH, Martin F. (1996): The Philosophical Inscription of Diogenes of Oinoanda. Wien.

SMITH, Martin F. (2000): Digging up Diogenes: New Epicurean texts from Oinoanda in Lycia. In: ERLER (2000), p. 64–75.

SMITH, Martin F. (2003): Supplement to Diogenes of Oinoanda. The Epicurean inscription (= La scuola di Epicuro Supplementi, 3). Napoli.

SMITH, Wesley D. (1982): Erasistratus' Dietetic Medicine. In: Bulletin of the History of Medicine 56, p. 398–409.

SOBEL, Hildegard (1990): Hygieia. Die Göttin der Gesundheit. Darmstadt.

SOLIN, Heikki (2013): Inschriftliche Wunderheilungsberichte aus Epidauros. In: Zeitschrift für antikes Christentum 17, p. 7–50.

STADEN, Heinrich von (1982): Hairesis and Heresy: the Case of Hairesis Iatrikai. In: MEYER, Ben F.; SANDERS, E. Paul (ed.): Jewish and Christian Self-definition. Vol. 3. Self-definition in the Graeco-Roman World. London, p. 76–100.

STADEN, Heinrich von (1989): Herophilos. The art of medicine in early Alexandria. Edition, translation and essays. Cambridge.

STADEN, Heinrich von (1990): Incurability and Hopelessness: The Hippocratic Corpus. In: POTTER, Paul; MALONEY, Gilles; DESAUTELS, Jacques (ed.): La maladie et les maladies dans la Collection hippocratique. Paris, p. 75–112.

STADEN, Heinrich von (1995): Anatomy as Rhetoric: Galen on dissection and persuasion. In: Journal of the History of Medicine and allied Sciences 50, p. 47–66.

STADEN, Peter J. van (1998): Jesus and Asklepios. In: Ekklesiastikos Pharos 80, p. 84–111.

STAFFORD, Emma J. (1998): Greek Cults of deified Abstractions. Diss. London.

STAMATU, Marion (2005): Fluch. In: LEVEN (2005), col. 303.

STANNARD, Jerry (1987): Herbal Medicine and Herbal Magic in Pliny's Time. In: PIGEAUD, Jackie; OROZ RETA, José. (ed.): Pline l'ancien, témoin de son temps. Salamanca, Nantes, p. 95–106.

STEGER, Florian (2000): Erinnern an Asklepios. Lektüre eines gegenwärtigen Mythos aus der antiken Medizin. In: JAGOW, Bettina von (ed.): Topographie der Erinnerung – Mythos im strukturellen Wandel. Würzburg, p. 19–39.

STEGER, Florian (2001): Rez. zu SCHULZE (1999). In: Gymnasium 108 (2001), p. 543–545.

STEGER, Florian (2004): Asklepiosmedizin. Medizinischer Alltag in der römischen Kaiserzeit (= Medizin, Gesellschaft und Geschichte Beiheft, 22). Stuttgart.

STEGER, Florian (2005a): Der Neue Asklepios Glykon. In: Medizinhistorisches Journal 40, p. 1–16.

STEGER, Florian (2005b): Wasser erfassen – Wasser wahrnehmen. Religiöse, soziale und medizinische Funktionen des Wassers: Kult und Medizin des Asklepios. In: Sylvelyn Hähner-Rombach (ed.): „Ohne Wasser ist kein Heil". Medizinische und kulturelle Aspekte der Nutzung von Wasser (= Medizin, Gesellschaft und Geschichte Beiheft, 25). Stuttgart, p. 33–43.

STEGER, Florian (2007): Patientengeschichte. Eine Perspektive für Quellen der Antiken Medizin? In: Sudhoffs Archiv 91, p. 230–238.

STEGER, Florian (2012): Asklepios in der Praxis. Medizinischer Alltag in der römischen Kaiserzeit. In: GERSTENGARBE, Sybille; KAASCH, Joachim; KAASCH, Michael; KLEINERT, Andreas und PARTHIER, Benno (ed.): Acta Historica Leopoldina 59. Stuttgart, p. 77–93.

STEGER, Florian (2016a): Asklepios. Medizin und Kult. Stuttgart.

STEGER, Florian (2016b): Aristides, Patient of Asclepius in Pergamum. In: RUSSELL, David A.; TRAPP, Michael; NESSELRATH, Heinz-Günther (ed.): Aelius Aristides. Selected Prose Hymns. Introduction, text, translation and interpretative essays (= Scripta ANtiquitatis Posterioris ad Ethicam Religionemque pertinentia, 29). Tübingen, p. 129–142.

STRATEN, Folkert T. van (1981): Gifts for the God. In: VERSNEL, Hendrik p. (ed.): Faith, Hope and Worship: Aspects of Religious Mentality in the Ancient World. Leiden, p. 65–151.

STROBEL, Karl (1993): Das Imperium Romanum im „3. Jahrhundert": Modell einer historischen Krise? Zur Frage mentaler Strukturen breiter Bevölkerungsschichten in der Zeit von Marc Aurel bis zum Ausgang des 3. Jh. n. Chr. (= Historia Einzelschriften, 75). Stuttgart.

STROHMAIER, Gotthard (1996): Die Rezeption und die Vermittlung: die Medizin in der byzantinischen und arabischen Welt. In: GRMEK (1996), p. 151–181.

STROHMAIER, Gotthard (1999): Avicenna. München.

SWAIN, Simon (1991): The Reliability of Philostratus's „Lives of the Sophists". In: Classical Antiquity 10, p. 148–163.

SWAIN, Simon (1996): Hellenism and Empire. Language, classicism, and power in the Greek world. AD 50–250. Oxford.

SZAIVERT, Wolfgang (2008): Kistophoren und die Münzbilder in Pergamon. In: Numismatische Zeitschrift 116–117, p. 29–43.

T

TABANELLI, Mario (1962): Gli ex-voto poliviscerali etrusci e romani. Storia, ritrovamento interpretazione. Firenze.

TEMKIN, Owsei (1991): Hippokrates in a World of Pagans and Christians. Baltimore, London.

TIELEMAN, Teun (2005): Pneumatiker. In: LEVEN (2005), col. 718–719.

TOMLINSON, Richard A. (1969): Two Buildings in the Sanctuaries of Asklepios. In: Journal of Hellenic Studies 89, p. 106–117.

TOMLINSON, Richard A. (1983): Epidauros. Austin (Texas).

TOTELIN, Laurence M. V. (2016): Pharmakopōlai. A re-evaluation of the sources. In: HARRIS (2016), p. 65–85.

TOTTI-GEMÜND, Maria (1998): Aretalogie des Imuthes-Asklepios (P. Oxy. 1381,64–145). In: GIRONE (1998), p. 169–193.

TOUWAIDE, Alain (1997): Galien et la Toxicologie. In: ANRW 37,2. Berlin, New York, p. 1887–1986.

TURFA, Jean M. (1994): Anatomical Votives and Italian Medical Tradition. In: SMALL, Jocelyn P.; DE PUMA, Richard D. (ed.): Murlo and the Etruscans. Art and society in ancient Etruria. Madison, p. 224–240.

U

URSIN, Frank (2014): Eusebeia und Asebeia als Bewertungskriterien von Herrschern bei Pausanias. In: Keryx 3, P. 55–68.

URSIN, Frank; STEGER, Florian; BORELLI, Claudia (2018): Katharsis of the skin. Peeling applications and agents of chemical peelings in Greek medical textbooks of Graeco-Roman antiquity. In: Journal of the European Academy of Dermatology and Venereology, https://doi.org/10.1111/jdv.15026.

V

VAN DER EIJK, Philip; HORSTMANSHOFF, H. F. J.; SCHRIJVERS, Petrus H. (ed.) (1995): Ancient Medicine in its socio-cultural context. 2 Vols. (= Clio Medica, 28). Amsterdam.

VAN GENNEP, Arnold (1909): Les rites de passage. Étude systématique des rites de la porte et du seuil, de l'hospitalité, de l'adoption, de la grossesse et de l'accouchement, de la naissance, de l'enfance, de la puberté, de l'initiation, de l'ordination, du couronnement, des fiançailles et du mariage, de funérailles, des saisons, etc. Paris.

VALLANCE, John T. (1990): The Lost Theory of Asclepiades of Bithynia. Oxford.

VALLANCE, John T. (1993): The Medical System of Asclepiades of Bithynia. In: ANRW II 37,1. Berlin; New York, p. 693–727.

VIDMAN, Ladislav (1970): Isis und Sarapis bei den Griechen und den Römern. Epigraphische Studien zur Verbreitung und zu den Trägern des ägyptischen Kultes. Berlin.

VLASTOS, Gregory (1948): Religion and Medicine in the Cult of Asclepius: a review article. In: Review of Religion 13, p. 269–290.

W

WACHT, Manfred (1999): Inkubation. In: Reallexikon für Antike und Christentum 18, p. 179–265.

WALDE, Christine (2001): Antike Traumdeutung und moderne Traumforschung. Düsseldorf, Zürich.

WALTON, Alice (1965): The Cult of Asklepios. New York (= reprint of the edition of 1894).

WEBER, Gregor (2000): Kaiser, Träume und Visionen in Prinzipat und Spätantike (= Historia Einzelschriften, 143). Stuttgart.

WEGNER, Max (1961): Asklepios. In: Hippokrates 32, p. 976–982.

WEINREICH, Otto (1909): Antike Heilungswunder. Untersuchungen zum Wunderglauben der Griechen und Römer (= Religionsgeschichtliche Versuche und Vorarbeiten, 8). Gießen.

WEISS, Peter (1982): Ein Altar für Gordian III., die älteren Gordiane und die Severer auf Aigeai (Kilikien). In: Chiron 12, p. 191–205.

WEISSER, Ursula. (1983): Ibn Sina und die Medizin des arabisch-islamischen Mittelalters – Alte und neue Urteile und Vorurteile. In: Medizinhistorisches Journal 18, p. 283–305.

WELLMANN, Max (1900): A. Cornelius Celsus. In: RE IV 1 (1900), col. 1882–1886.

WESCH-KLEIN, Gabriele (1998): Soziale Aspekte des römischen Heerwesens in der Kaiserzeit (= HABES, 28). Stuttgart.

WICKKISER, Bronwen L. (2008): Asklepios, medicine, and the politics of healing in fifth-century Greece. Between craft and cult. Baltimore (Md.).

WICKKISER, Bronwen L. (2010): Banishing Plague. Asklepios, Athens, and the great plague reconsidered. In: JENSEN, Jesper T. (ed.): Aspects of ancient Greek cult. Context, ritual and iconography (= Aarhus studies in Mediterranean antiquity, 8). Aarhus, p. 55–65.

WIDE, Sam (1973): Lakonische Kulte. Darmstadt.

WIEDEMANN, Thomas (1995): Emperors and Gladiators. London, New York.

WIEMER, Hans-Ulrich (1997): Iulian. In: CLAUSS (1997), p. 334–341.

WILAMOWITZ MOELLENDORFF, Ulrich von (1886): Isyllos von Epidauros. Berlin.

WILDUNG, Dieter (1975): Asklepios. In: LÄ. Vol. 1, col. 472–473.

WILDUNG, Dieter (1977): Heilschlaf. In: LÄ. Vol. 2, col. 1101–1102.

WILMANNS, Juliane C. (1995): Der Sanitätsdienst im Römischen Reich. Eine sozialgeschichtliche Studie zum römischen Militärsanitätswesen nebst einer Prosopographie des Sanitätspersonals (= Medizin der Antike, 2). Hildesheim.

WITSCHEL, Christian (1999): Krise – Rezession – Stagnation? Der Westen des Römischen Reiches im 3. Jahrhundert n. Chr. Frankfurt/M.

WITTERN, Renate (1979): Die Unterlassung ärztlicher Hilfeleistung in der griechischen Medizin der klassischen Zeit. In: Münchener Medizinische Wochenschrift 121, p. 731–734.

WITTERN, Renate (1995): Die Anfänge der Anatomie im Abendland. In: SCHNALKE, Thomas (ed.): Natur im Bild. Erlangen, p. 21–51.

WITTERN, Renate (1998a): Die Antike in Mittelalter und Renaissance: Das Beispiel Anatomie. In: Nachrichtenblatt der deutschen Gesellschaft für Geschichte der Medizin, Naturwissenschaft und Technik 48, p. 146–159.

WITTERN, Renate (1998b): Gattungen im Corpus Hippocraticum. In: KULLMANN/ALTHOFF/ASPER (1998), p. 17–36.

WITTERN, Renate (1999): Kontinuität und Wandel in der Medizin des 14. bis 16. Jahrhunderts am Beispiel der Anatomie. In: HAUG, Walter (ed.): Mittelalter und frühe Neuzeit: Übergänge, Umbrüche und Neuansätze (= Fortuna vitrea, 16). Stuttgart, p. 550–571.

WOLFF, Eberhard (1998a): Perspektiven der Patientengeschichtsschreibung. In: PAUL/SCHLICH (1998), p. 311–334.

WOLFF, Eberhard (1998b): Perspectives on Patients' History: Methodological Considerations on the Example of Recent German-Speaking Literature. In: Canadian Bulletin for Medical History 15, p. 207–228.

Z

ZEPPEZAUER, Dorothea (2013): Warum wirken Wunder? Die Sprache der Ärzte im Traum. In: Zeitschrift für antikes Christentum 17, p. 143–159.

ZIEGENAUS, Oskar; LUCA, Gioia de (1981): Das Asklepieion: Die Kultbauten aus römischer Zeit an der Ostseite des heiligen Bezirks (= Altertümer von Pergamon XI,3). Berlin, New York.

ZIEGLER, Ruprecht (1994): Aigeai, der Asklepioskult, das Kaiserhaus der Decier und das Christentum. In: Tyche 9, p. 187–212.

ZIETHEN, Gabriele (1994): Heilung und römischer Kaiserkult. In: Sudhoffs Archiv 78, p. 171–191.

V.3 – Picture credits

Fig. 1:   Serpent of Asclepius, mosaic, Lindau (Germany). Photo: Florian Steger.
Fig. 2:   London, British Museum. Medallion of Antoninus Pius. PENSO (1984),
            p. 12.
Fig. 3:   Epidauros, Museum No. 813 and Athens, National Archaeological Museum
            No. 266, 1347. Photo: Museum.
Fig. 4:   Athens, National Archaeological Museum No. 1402. From Luku. Marble,
            height 51 cm. Photo: akg-images / De Agostini Picture Lib.
Fig. 5:   Cos, Archaeological Museum. Without inventory number.
            Photo: Florian Steger.
Fig. 6:   HART (2000), fig. in appendix.
Fig. 7:   HART (2000), p. 116.
Fig. 8:   Cos, Asclepieion: View from the entrance toward the three-level terrace.
            Photo: Florian Steger.
Fig. 9 a/b: Rome, Tiber Island. Photo: Giovanni Rubeis.
Fig. 10:   Giovanni Battista Piranesi: Vedute di Roma, ca. 1780. Photo: Wellcome
            Collection.
Fig. 11:   Epidaurus, plan of Asclepieion. IAKOVIDIS (1985), p. 131.
Fig. 12:   Cos, plan of Asclepieion. KRUG (1993), p. 161 fig. 73.
Fig. 13 a/b: Pergamum, plan of Asclepieion. RADT (1999), p. 221 figs. 167 and 168.
Fig. 14 a/b: Pergamum, Asclepieion. RADT (1999), p. 229 figs. 175 and 176.
Fig. 15:   Cos, Asclepieion, entrance: residential buildings. Photo: Florian Steger.
Fig. 16:   Cos, Asclepieion, entrance: residential buildings and bath.
            Photo: Florian Steger.
Fig. 17:   Cos, Asclepieion, view from the intermediate level (between middle and
            upper terrace) to the middle and lower terrace. Photo: Florian Steger.
Fig. 18:   Cos, Asclepieion, upper terrace, Doric temple of Asclepius.
            Photo: Florian Steger.
Fig. 19:   Cos, Asclepieion, upper terrace, Doric temple of Asclepius.
            Photo: Florian Steger.
Fig. 20:   Epidaurus. IG IV^2 1.126 = SIG III 1170. Photo: Museum.

V.4 – Index of persons and places

V.5 – Subject index

anatomical votives 37, 91, 93, 137

apodyterium 83 f.

archiater 30, 134

architecture 65 f., 70, 89, 109, 136

Asclepieion 19, 38, 41, 44 f., 47 f., 50 f., 53, 60, 62, 66–83, 90–96, 105, 109, 114, 121 f., 124 f., 131, 137

bread 123, 125, 127

caldarium 83 f.

capsarius 35

celery 123, 125 f.

cheese 85, 123, 125 f.

cock 85, 98, 152

Corpus Hippocraticum 27, 139

curse tablets 56

dietetics 28

dill 123, 127, 131

disease 33, 37, 45, 47, 55, 66, 91, 94, 97, 102 f.

dog 19, 41

dogmatists 20, 22–24, 133

dream 16, 20, 38, 56, 85–91, 95, 98–102, 107–118, 129 f., 137

egg 55, 79, 117

empiricists 20–24, 27, 133, 134

frigidarium 84

healing, miracle 5, 9–20, 29–31, 35, 37–43, 45, 47–79, 81–110, 113, 117, 125, 128 f., 131–138

health 9, 15, 28 f., 33, 35, 37, 40, 42, 56 f., 66–71, 82, 91, 96 f., 101, 104, 111, 114–116, 118, 124, 128, 132, 135–138

Hieroi Logoi 87, 106–109, 118 f.

honey 98, 123, 125, 127

humoral pathology 20, 24, 27, 134

Iamata 57 f., 94, 96, 98

Iamatika 95, 151

incubation 20, 73, 76, 78, 81, 84–90, 109 f., 121, 129, 137

inscription 10, 14–16, 19, 30, 32, 37 f., 47, 53, 56–58, 60, 62, 64, 79, 81 f., 92 f., 94, 96, 98, 102, 105, 120–122, 125, 129–132, 135, 137–139

laconicum 84

lettuce 123, 125 f.

magic 9 f., 12, 15, 17, 29, 54–57, 94, 135

medicus 17, 29 f., 34, 38 f., 49

methodists 20, 22–24, 27, 127, 133

midwife 30, 135

military 9, 25 f., 32, 33 f., 62, 134, 135

milk 114, 123, 125–127

mustard 123, 127

myrrh 126, 131

mythos 140, 157

neokorate 60

Oath of Hippocrates 30 f.

oil 35, 83, 88, 111, 123, 127

Omphalos 53, 59

onion 129–131

papyrus 95 f., 139

patient 12, 13, 16, 20, 22, 25 f., 30 f., 34, 36, 40, 43, 54, 58, 65 f., 70 f., 73, 82–88, 91, 97, 101–117, 119–125, 127 f., 131, 133 f., 136–138

pepper 129–132

physician 9, 12–15, 17, 19–36, 48, 54 f., 57, 61, 65 f., 84, 87 f., 92, 97–99, 101, 103, 105, 110, 113–120, 134 f., 137

piscina 84

plague 17, 27, 37–39, 45, 47, 55, 93, 114, 118, 136

plaster 127

pneumatists 20

propylon 53, 71, 78

purgative 115